From Surgeon to Shaman

Living a Directed Life

Kenneth Hawley Hamilton, MD, CM, FACS

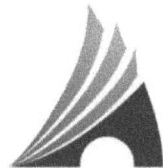

BookLocker

Saint Petersburg, Florida

Healing of Persons Exceptional

www.hopehealing.org

Copyright © 2022 by Kenneth Hawley Hamilton, M.D.

ISBN: 978-0-9725760-1-7

First Edition

Printed on acid-free paper.

BookLocker.com, Inc.
2022

Earlier books:

SoulCircling, The Journey to the Who (Hope Healing Publications, 2002)

The H.O.P.E. Story, with Joyce O. Murphy, R.N. (Hope Healing Publications, 2007)

Table of Contents

Prologue

A stranger's strange insight

When I was four, a total stranger walked up to me as I was walking the familiar roads of Forest Hills, Long Island. I was wont to take these walks because I liked them in this quiet suburb of New York City. I knew all of the roads that led to my home, and my mother was never worried about my wanderings around town. A woman I did not recognize came up to me and asked me if I knew where I lived. To my "Yes", she asked me if I would show her my way home. That was okay with me and I remember her taking my left hand in her right hand and saying, "Show me."

I took her to my home. She asked if she could talk to my mother, and I agreed. We walked up to the front door. She rang the doorbell, and when my mother opened the door, she asked my mother if I was I her son. To my mother's "Yes," she said, "Please take very good care of him… he is very important to the world." My mother thanked her. She said "Goodbye," turned, and left. I never saw her again. My mother repeated this important instruction several times during my very young years. (She knew what she was doing… making sure that the planted seed became a tree.)

Dedication

This book is dedicated to my dear friend, Tom (Thomas E.) Flagg, who showed me so much about nature, helping me appreciate what life was all about. We met in the eastern Adirondacks where I summered from infancy until I was seventeen and headed for college. Tom lived with his widowed mother about a mile across the valley from my paternal grandmother and one of her daughters, for whom she worked keeping house. She brought us together. Magic happened and Tom and I are fast friends to this day... gratitude abides.

Acknowledgements

I wish to acknowledge twelve people who, more than any others, played a significant role in shaping my life: Amy Gordon Hamilton, Jim McAlister, Earl Nightingale, Barry Wood, Bernie Siegel, Gerry Jampolsky, Bob Snowman, Margot Taylor Fanger, Ruth Dullea, Dennise Whitley, and Sid Russell. Are they "teachers?" Are they "coaches?" Are they "guides?" Is there one word that includes all three designations? I'll leave you to figure out that answer for yourself. In addition, hundreds of H.O.P.E. Group participants – "H.O.P.E.rs" – in over 5,000 H.O.P.E. Group meetings helped mature the gifts of the twelve. Each of these H.O.P.E.rs demonstrated clearly how the will to live fought the cancer in their bodies supporting themselves and the people around them. In the words of one great old H.O.P.E.r, "I may have cancer, but it don't have me."

I begin with my beloved Aunt, Amy Gordon Hamilton, who was a spiritual guide from my earliest years. She was my father's younger sister who had to have an emergency hysterectomy for hemorrhage when she was a teenager, a century ago (I tell the story behind it on p. 25.) She knew by the social rules of the day that her operation made it impossible for her to marry, because she could never give a man children. When she was a student at Bryn Mawr College, she found social work to be a powerful call. She went on to become an assistant Dean in the New York School of Social Work of Columbia University with the well-earned reputation for being a "giant" in the realm of social casework.

Wise to the ways of the times, Amy Gordon chose to be known by her middle name, Gordon. Her pen name became "A. Gordon Hamilton". She told me that when she would attend a conference there would be men who would express surprise when they met, saying, "So you're A. Gordon Hamilton. I always thought you were a man."

I used to visit her in New York to be present to her wisdom. At one of these visits, I was telling her all about my experiences with God. She said that the God of her Christian Science family was not her God, which may have made her an atheist, but she loved human beings. Those words went to my core. I recall her voice and her apartment where she shared her experience of loving human beings in their struggles

Dennise Whitley was the first person I met when I went to Stephens Memorial Hospital to be interviewed for a position as a staff General Surgeon. She met me with a charming smile and an openness that introduced her and that discovered my reason for standing at the open door to her office. I felt welcome in that instant. She made me feel welcome to the whole hospital, and her nurturing nature led me to use her as a ready resource for thoughts, opinions, smiles and laughs as my relationship with that fine hospital benefited and grew. She became a fast friend and supporter, for whom I feel great gratitude that endures richly through the next fifty years.

My practice manager, Jim McAlister – an intuitive guide if there ever was one – was the first and only person to whom I owned a family heritage of anger. I had come under a lot of stress back in 1973 as president of the hospital staff and a growing influx of new staff members, coupled with a stunning process that summarizes where I have been my whole life... every time I got to the stop sign at the end of the street where I had my office, there was traffic there going my way, and I would have to wait for all of those cars to get past that stop sign before I could join the queue. This was not a random event, but something that happened every time I got to that particular stop sign for the preceding three months. My family legacy of angry men grew and grew until finally I complained to Jim. His response was, "Ken, I got an *"INSIGHT"* tape from the Nightingale–Conant Corporation last week and Earl was talking about something that I think applies here. I'll loan you this tape on penalty of death if you don't give it back." He asked me if I was familiar with Nightingale. I was. When I was stationed in Germany, I used to listen to Nightingale in his five-minute weekly Insight segment about his experiences with life.

In the *INSIGHT* tape, Earl described what he called, "The Law of Correspondence." That law said that the attitudes you see in the world around you reflect the attitudes you project into that world. If you don't like what you're seeing, remember that you chose that attitude at a time when it worked, and if you don't like it you can change it; for all attitudes are chosen. That piece of advice stunned me. I knew I had a choice I could make. As I was getting in my car to go home that day, I found myself saying to myself, "Take it easy Ken." Needless to say, I had a touch of anxiety five times before I got to that stop sign, and each time I repeated, "Take it easy, Ken," I felt more comfortable. I snuck up to that stop sign with my eyes nearly shut, concerned that I would not see another car there. It was quite an effort, but when I opened my eyes wide there was only one car in sight, and I was sitting in it! That changed my life forever.

I subscribed to those *INSIGHT* tapes. Today, I have 22 years of those monthly, 60-minute tapes in my basement. Every one of them holds four 15-minute interviews of specialists in human development. The last segment was always Earl, who, in my opinion, was the world's greatest student of success... "the progressive realization of a worthy ideal". I listened to each one of them several times before the next one came. I have passed on the experience in every one of those tapes to my patients, and it was always received with gratitude. It made my reputation for kindness, concern, and respect for all my patients... helping them "get on with their lives".

Earl had a three – part gift for everyone: a Formula; a Gold Mine; and a Word. The Formula was the universal spiritual perception – "We become what we think about most." The Gold Mine is that which does the thinking – the Mind. The key to each of the rooms of the Gold Mine is one Word, "Attitude". He went on to say that The Law of Correspondence is a spiritual law that is to be found in every spiritual tradition in the world. Each of those monthly tapes had four presentations, the first three of which were made by people known to Earl, and the fourth was Earl, himself. I used the tape player in my car to listen to the most recent tape every time I drove somewhere... I loved the experience.

The result was that I realized I was onto a healing psychology that I had never encountered in my medical career. However, I had learned in the first class in pathology in my second year at McGill University Faculty of Medicine that the most important quality of a McGill physician beyond always doing her or his professional best was to be able to promise her/his patients that s-he would do everything in her/his power to help that patient get on with her or his life. I was learning from Earl and company how to be able to fulfill that promise to my patients. Twelve years later, the changes that had come about in me would lead me to Barry Wood, MD

The social worker at my hospital introduced us. She was a good friend, who I used to visit frequently in her hospital office. One day, she told me that she was going to take a sabbatical and get a graduate degree in psychology. That rang a bell in me, and I had been thinking pretty much the same thing. She said, "I don't think you would like that. You would have to take two full semesters of mathematics." Yes, she had guessed that I was not particularly fond of advanced mathematics, so I asked her if she had an alternative. Her reply was, "consider getting 'tutorial counseling'." In response to my query about it, she suggested that I work with a medical professional to learn counseling, suggesting a psychiatrist who was as specialized in helping humans correct disorders of their psyche as I was specialized in surgery. I accepted that. I asked her if she had someone in mind, and I knew that her "No" was a lie. Two days later she gave me a Post-it with his name and telephone number and advised that I call him and see if the music was there. I did, and it was.

Barry was a complex human being with board certifications in internal medicine and psychiatry. He was an ordained Episcopal minister with a doctorate in theology. He was the adult child of an alcoholic mother. He was, himself, a recovering alcoholic. He had "come out" of a straight marriage and stood for his ex-wife when she remarried after their divorce. He got me participating in twelve-step group meetings, where vitally important component was that there was no "facilitator" to "run" such a meeting. It was all about surrendering one's ego to the power of a much greater Being

When we were still working together on a weekly basis, Barry was admitted to hospital with rectal bleeding. He was found to have a cancer of the colon that a surgical colleague of mine resected, but he did not regain intestinal function postoperatively. He was obstructed. Re-exploration revealed the diffuse spread of the malignancy throughout his abdominal cavity with one focus of obstruction. His surgeon bypassed that blockage and the oncologists started him on chemotherapy. While he was still in the hospital after his second operation, he asked his partner to bring him the Sunday *New York Times*. As was his wont, he went directly to the book reviews, and, to his delight, he read the review of Bernie Siegel's first book, *Love Medicine and Miracles* (HarperCollins 1986), and sent his partner off to buy a copy of it. He read it avidly, and when he got home with his intestines working, he called Bernie and said, "I want to come down and see you." Bernie replied, "I'm busy, and you are postop. I have 30 minutes and they're yours." Bernie conveyed to Barry the nature of his work in that 3–minute gift. They never saw each other but stayed in touch. When Barry and I started working together again, he said "I never tell my patients what to do, but I strongly recommend that you get the book, read it, and get in touch with the author."

I did as I was told, ordering it on my way home. It arrived two days later. I had it read by the end of the weekend, and on the following Monday my social worker friend gave me a catalog for Interface workshops in Watertown, Massachusetts. She thought I might like Bernie's work, and right there was a weekend workshop with Bernie Siegel! It was a weekend where I had three days off call. I signed up for it and heard him describe in depth his Exceptional Cancer Patients (ECaP) Groups and guided imagery. The work of these groups was based on the nurturance of healthy, healing attitudes... all shared through the loving nature of the good Dr. Siegel. Bernie and I established a friendship then that endures to this day.

At that conference, I mentioned to the hosts my appreciation of the value of supportive groups. Faculty members told me that a psychiatrist from the West Coast would be coming in a month to give his experience with what he called "Attitudinal Healing". That psychiatrist turned out to be Gerald G Jampolsky, MD. Gerry had suffered emotional abuse growing up because he was dyslexic, and his family called him "dummy" in a time when nobody knew anything about dyslexia. As is so common in such confusing situations, humans resort to attack behavior in order to help the other overcome dysfunctional behavior.

Today we know that to insult a child is a form of abandonment. H.O.P.E. Group work has shown me that all forms of abandonment comprise key factors in the development of narcissistic personality disorders.

Gerry was introduced to *A Course In Miracles* (ACIM) by Judith Skutch Whitson who asked him for his opinion of its psychology. His response is notable: "You don't want me reviewing this. It's Christian. I am a Jew, and furthermore I am an atheist." Judy's reply was to tell Gerry that he was a very good psychologist/psychiatrist, and because Gerry was Gerry, they wanted his opinion as to the quality of the text. He submitted to their request and got about halfway through the Course text when it hit him "one upside the head." He said to himself (as he has told me): "Gerry, this is your way home. Physician heal thyself." The effect was instantaneous. He came to love himself, forgiving himself for all of his rages, anger, cruel behavior, and complex addictions – instantaneously. Gerry and I established a friendship during his workshop, and it endures to this day.

Bob Snowman and I had known each other for years before he found peace and love in the H.O.P.E. Group I had started in my surgical practice for my cancer patients. Bob was a newspaper person whose articles were always well-written and informative. He brought a fine writer's eye to the H.O.P.E. Group who welcomed him as a friend dealing with cancer. He died suddenly one morning standing in the front door to his home. A neighbor saw him collapse and called 911, but Bob could not be resuscitated. He is missed.

Margot Taylor Fanger and I met at a conference in Kansas. It was a meeting that had all of the hallmarks of the latest installment of sharing many past lives. Margot was an A.C.S.W. doing social work in a Boston suburb. In addition, she was a Master Neurolinguistic Programmer, and very wise in the ways of human beings. It is no coincidence that I am the nephew of one of the Social Work giants, my father's younger sister, Amy Gordon Hamilton. I know the language of Social Work. Margot was a gem of a human being and an associate professor in the School of Social Work affiliated with Columbia University, New York.

She participated in H.O.P.E. in many ways, one of which was working with me to develop a certificated training program. She had a clear focus on H.O.P.E. and in regular visits to H.O.P.E. she helped me develop it into the solid program it is today. She advised me never to say to a person, "How can I help you?" because it contained two false assumptions: first, assuming that the other *wanted* help; and second, my *ability to provide that help*. Instead, she taught me the indirect, subjunctive way of asking, "What would you like to have happen?" She showed me how the work of a social worker served humans challenged by life in all its many manifestations. I have taken all of that which she taught as a contextual framework for the work that H.O.P.E. provides.

Ruth Dullea was a patient of mine who had a recurrent cancer. She was the mother of Dennise Whitley who was the first person I met when I entered Stephens Memorial Hospital to see if it was where I would like to have a surgical career. We clicked then, and the click holds today. She has been a faithful, motherly supporter of the program.

The last person in my list of acknowledgments was a recovering alcoholic, Sid Russell. He presented in my surgical practice with a small basal cell skin cancer on his face that I removed. He then came with hoarseness that revealed a tumor on a vocal cord an otolaryngologist friend of mine removed successfully. He then came to me with rectal bleeding and barium enema revealed a small cancer in the descending colon. However, blood tests suggested that it had spread to his liver, and at exploration and resection of the involved segment of his intestine I found metastatic nodules in both lobes of his liver… incurable. Sid should have lived only one and one-half years, but he lived for three full years. He was the least anonymous alcoholic in my community in rural Maine. He was active in AA, and loved the country, canoeing, fishing, and being with friends. He had that "recovery" way about him, which was straightforward, honest, and nurturing. His presence in any H.O.P.E. Group meeting was a joy. His style was the style of a commercial pilot who used to fly a DC 3 over The Hump in the eastern end of the Himalayas resupplying the Chinese war effort from 1942 to 1945. Alcoholism was common to those pilots, and Sid's alcoholism continued when he got back to America and lasted until he found AA.

Sid was bright, clever, loving, kind, honest… qualities of a recovering alcoholic. It was beautifully manifest in his visits to the local H.O.P.E. group, of which he was a member. When I hold Sid's experience up to Barry's, I find resources to work with people who have addictions of virtually any kind.

As the result of working with these individuals in H.O.P.E. Groups, I acknowledge, and am deeply grateful, to all these wonderful people with whom I have had the privilege of working in weekly two-hour meetings.

Finally, I wish to acknowledge the existence of that which is known as "Aleph[iv]" On the one hand, it is the first letter of three Semitic alphabets. On the other, it is said to be the timeless source of our infinite, *conscious* universe. I have shared several inexplicable things that happened in my life, all of which lead me to an appreciation for Aleph, the Mystery behind all life.

Epigraphs

- Tao Te Ching
  The Tao that can be trodden
  is not the enduring and unchanging Tao.
  The name that can be named
  is not the enduring and unchanging name

  (Conceived of as) having no name,
  it is the Originator of heaven and earth;
  (Conceived of as) having a name,
  it is the Mother of all things
    —Lao Tzu (J. Legge Translator), (Sacred Books of the East,
    Vol 39) [1891]

- "I know something about you that you don't know I know, and aren't
  you going to be surprised when you find it out what it is."
    —Milton H. Erickson, MD

- "Another world is not only possible, she is on her way.
  On a quiet day, I can hear her breathing."
    —Arundhati Roy

- Holy listening—to listen another's soul into life, into a condition of
  disclosure and discovery, may be almost the greatest service that
  any human being ever performs for another.
    —Douglas V. Steere (1901-1995)

- "Hope is the source and spring of all the alchemies of
  transformation, the greatest treasure of the heart and mind, the
  philosopher's stone that transmutes agony and tragedy into new life.
  Never abandon hope, or you abandon your closest and most helpful
  guide, the friend."
    —Rumi

- "There is a road, no simple highway
  Between the dawn and the dark of night
  And if you go no one may follow
  That path is for your steps alone.

  Ripple in still water
  When there is no pebble tossed
  Nor wind to blow"
    —Grateful Dead Songwriters: Gerry Garcia, Robert Hunter

- Listen and Witness
  Listen to the song in my heart
  Listen to the song in my heart
  Listen to my heartsong.
  Listen to my heart song.
  Listen to the song in my heart

  Witness the beauty of my dance.
  Witness the beauty of my dance.
  Witness my beauty dance.
  Witness my beauty dance.
  Witness the beauty of my dance.

  Listen to the cry of my soul.
  Listen to the cry of my soul.
  Listen to my soul cry.
  Listen to my soul cry.
  Listen to the cry of my soul.
    —Richard Lawrance

Foreword

(Author's note: My wife wrote this piece about two years after I had taken training in shamanic soul retrieval given by Sandra Ingerman, who was then active in the work of The Foundation for Shamanic Studies (https://www.shamanism.org/). My wife wrote this out of her own initiative and gave it to me shortly after she finished it. This woke me up to what was happening, and I wrote the first piece called "From Surgeon to Shaman" in May of 1999, setting an intention for the next nine years. I have learned that setting an intention is, for me, a spiritual process that will materialize when the best time comes.)

February 1998

My Life as the Wife of a Surgeon turned Shaman.

I made a good catch marrying a budding doctor just out of medical school. The fact my mother-in-law didn't hesitate to point out; and he, her wonderful son, was obviously bedazzled by my sex-appeal since I was from Scandinavia, and everybody knew love = sex was rampant in those countries. Besides, I wore a very small bikini. Luckily, I love my man for other reasons than his earning capacity, which didn't come into play 'til many years later. First there was internship, residency, specialty training with very little money and a surprise daughter eleven months after the wedding and two years later a son. A perfect family. Yes.

Being the wife of the doctor in those days was – shall we say – challenging. The doctor is considered a god by many including himself. How can you argue with a man who was busy, so very busy <u>saving lives</u>? I learned and the kids learned to live with this basically wonderful man who was boss-God and wage earner and often absent.

The years passed, life went on and then slowly a whole other side of husband/father started to emerge. He worked on developing intuition, sensitivity, patience. Slowly at first, then faster, a new husband appeared, spiritual with many fancy flights of the imagination (in my opinion). He retired from the "cut and cure" school of thought and is now helping people to use alternative ways to heal.

Marvelous, you say. Lucky you, you think.

Well, wait a minute, where is the man I married, to whom I adapted so well over 20 or so years? I don't remember getting a divorce and joining souls with <u>this</u> touchy-feely person. I was aghast, should I leave now or did this mean had to change, too? Me, who always has been earth bound, sensible, and realistic, in short, pretty near perfect!

The most incredible thing is happening. By brainwashing, osmosis, whatever, in small ways, his attitude is corrupting me, undermining my staunch no-nonsense self. Understand, I shall never become one with the universe in this life, but if I could survive his transformation – I still kind of love him – I can't be all I used to be, probably I am more.

Jonna M. Hamilton

Preface

There you have it. My wife's words in her foreword describe what happened to me and her when I was told that the work that I was doing in H.O.P.E. groups was quite similar to the work of the American shaman, Michael Harner, PhD, who created The Foundation for Shamanic Studies... it focused on that part of our being called the soul. I was strongly advised to read his book, The Way of the Shaman (HarperOne, 1990).. I followed that advice and was delighted to see that the work I was doing was like the work that had been going on for 30,000 years.

I am an avid reader of nonfiction and was disturbed by the early 17th century decision by the French Rationalists, of whom René Descartes was one, who decided that the soul did not exist, because its existence could not be "scientifically proven." When I became familiar with shamanic practices, it was clear to me that they dealt with the very thing that Descartes and his friends said could not exist. For me, my soul is the non-physical essence of *who* I am. My ego is the director – what I have come to call the "First Mate" – of my physical being: my "what". As I examined the work that I was doing in H.O.P.E. Groups, I literally helped people remember that they were spiritual beings – souls – living in a human body on a divine assignment... that which Earl Nightingale called a "worthy ideal". He went on to say that the progressive realization of that worthy ideal was "the essence of success."

The purpose of this book, my autobiography, is to encourage people to see themselves as anything but accidental products of an inanimate process. It has been 20 years since my wife wrote the words of the Foreword... 10 years after the first H.O.P.E. Group came into existence. That process can be taught and reproduced. I, personally, have over 5000 H.O.P.E. Group meetings in my experience, and have trained over 100 people in that "H.O.P.E. Group" process.

The process is not one of trying to fix something that is broken but one of sharing experience that helps people recognize the resources they were born with in order to fulfill a greater purpose in living. This a matter of putting life into the loving space called "compassion". Both the joy and the suffering can be... indeed be... held in the great forgiving field of compassion. Hear the words of the great 13th c. Persian poet, Jalal al-Din Rumi:

> "Out beyond ideas of wrongdoing and rightdoing, there is a field. I'll meet you there. When the soul lies down in that grass, the world is too full to talk about. Ideas, language, even the phrase 'each other' doesn't make any sense."
> — Coleman Barks (trans.)

You may ask, "does it have limitations?" The only limitation that I know about is that its value has not been applied widely enough to help us discover our true spiritual nature. I have written this book to share my experience with humanity to use as its members see fit. I have realized it is very important to be circumspect about giving advice... going so far as to discourage people from following thought patterns that make it possible to say, "How can I help you?" This implies that they need help in the first place and that I can provide it in the second place. Instead, consider Rumi's field and how you can create that space and invite another to join you there.

My question of anyone and everyone is: "What would you like to have happen in your life?"

And was I surprised when I found out that the question applied to me! I thought I was done with the whole thing a year ago... nobody interested in taking the H.O.P.E. business to the larger audience. "Me?" I asked Life. "Yup," says she, breaking my right hip in the neck of the femur! For no reasonable reason, I chose to tough it out overnight with the help of Aleve, and get to Stephens Hospital by ambulance the next morning. There I found that I was to have a Swedish-trained orthopedic surgeon who said, "You're lucky you have me... as opposed to your countryman who was on call yesterday, making you recover for four months by suturing the prosthesis in place. I'm going to cement that prosthesis in place and you'll be up walking tomorrow." He was true to his word, and I was home in three days!

During this precious time, a dozen people I'd worked with came to visit – separately – and every one of them reminded me of the wonderful way I cared for my patients. That was my passion that I'd found in second year of McGill

Medicine, when the pathology professor told the class: "Always do your professional best, and, more importantly, promise your patients that you'll do everything in your power to help them get on with their lives."

What a reminder from Life that she was not done with me! Today we need to hear more professionals say to those who suffer that we can and will do everything in our power to help them get on with their lives. What I first heard in 1962 became a promise to all I served... even now that I am well into the ninth decade of my life... I shall spend the rest of my time here on Mother Earth helping Her get on with Her life.

Introduction

Greetings... and thank you for coming to visit me, and to hear me tell you the story of my life – my experience with life that started UN-conventionally. "Life" kept on happening along its course with me that gave me pause to consider that I wasn't living "conventionally." Something gave me the sense that there really isn't any life we can call "conventional," and when I heard Earl Nightingale define success as "the progressive realization of a worthy ideal," he went on to say that everyone of us is born with just such a "worthy ideal", and Life gives everyone all the resources needed to identify and serve it. My career as a surgeon comprised a lot of listening to the stories of other human's lives... revealing to me the preciousness of every human being's story, for no two of them are alike.

There's a story in this that I wish to share , not because I want anyone to think I'm an expert who knows the way home, but that YOU are the expert born with the gifts of genes and environment that are an experience of value to everyone, especially that One who gave you this life and its assignment. I shall introduce you to the teachers I have had, and how they have contributed to this life I'm living. I shall share with you how I see you as a one-of-a-kind work of art... promised this life at the beginning of time... yes, we know now when time began. We know that both finite matter and infinite consciousness were there in that incredible moment.

I shall share with you what I consider to be my heritage... aspects of my present life that I have been led to see come from way back before Kenneth Hawley Hamilton was conceived. As the *shaman* in me has come to know, my spiritual guide is my soul, and, regardless of any arguments to the contrary, it has lived through many lifetimes as a human being. I have become aware of those lifetimes throughout my present life, and I have the clear sense that they have had a great bearing on how this life I am living has unfolded.

I shall share with you how I learned of the work that leads to this wonderful knowledge. Finally, I'll share with you the words of Peter Kingsley near the end of a masterpiece called *Reality* (The Golden Sufi Center; April 1, 2004). I hope to invite you to see life as a gift from Life, itself, the source of love, creativity, compassion, and kindness, all the while acknowledging the presence of the dark side of it all.

I shall share with you how I came to be aware that we are tripartite beings that are designed to work together to create a volume of unique experience in the Annals of the Universe.

I invite you to join me in an adventure that could not have been possible for ordinary souls like you and me until some 50-odd years ago. Let fear become awareness and anger become presence, and come along with me. I shall take you to my experience with Aleph, that "point outside of time and space" so richly covered in Paulo Coelho's autobiographical account – *Aleph* – of his 2006 Trans-Siberian rail journey of 9,288 kilometers. His experience with Aleph gave me a deeper appreciation of the mystical elements in my own life... I am quite certain most, if not all of you, will recall similar mysterious times in your lives.

Before we go any further, please go back to the quote from the *Tao Te Ching* that I listed first in the epigraph page. Yes, my friend, we are parts of a Mystery, and I offer you my story as an example... knowing that yours is also part of the Mystery. Come with me, starting with my experience with the three elements that comprise the Being of every human: Ego, Soul, and Spirit.

Chapter 1:
My Heritage

A Magyar Scot

What those two words say is my social and genetic heritage: Hungarian and Scot... in short, my mother and my father. My mother's mother was a Magor, which is a name that dates to earliest Hungarian origins: the two legendary ancestors of today's Hungarians were Hunor and Magor. My mother told me that she was descended from an offspring of Attila the Hun named Magor. Doing a little research showed me that Attila was a descendent of Magor, not the other way around

There is a history of the Magor people that my mother was fond of repeating... all of the Magor women look alike and the men do not look like the women but there is only one man in any generation who will have a son who will have a son to carry on the name. The similarities of the women are their handsome beauty, their faintly olive-tinged skin, their wavy, dark–brown hair, a certain prominence of jaw that was attractive and appealing, and striking yellow–brown eyes.

My mother had an experience in Europe in the 1920s that brings life to what I have just told you. She and a Magor cousin traveled to Europe... including Hungary... for obvious reasons. In Budapest, a Magor family member held a dinner for the two Magor women who looked like sisters. During the dinner, the two Canadians sat on either side of one man whom they did not know, and, across from them was another man who could not take his eyes off the two women. At the end of the meal this man spoke to the host and got his permission to meet the two Canadians. He begged forgiveness for his rudeness in staring at them both, but if they would be so kind as to come to his family home, he would show them why he stared at them. The host approved of this; so, the two Magor women went to this man's home the following day.

They got out of the taxi and as they were walking up to the front door it opened and the butler said, "Come in..." no request for identification. They entered and stood for a moment in the front hall where the owner greeted them, telling them that he wanted to show them why they had so fascinated him. He turned and opened the door to a large banquet hall that was lined with portraits of the men and women who had lived there for generations. All the women looked just like my mother and her cousin. The host did not have to say anything; he simply swung his arm around, waited a moment, then told them how he was so fascinated meeting another one of their old, old tribe. Today, my sister, who looks like our mother, has a daughter who has the Magor women's look. My sister recognized the Magor in her daughter and gave her "Magor" as a middle name. The Hungarian descendants of Magor seem to share a common DNA to this day.

My Scot heritage goes back a very long time because I grew up hearing much about that side of me. I never knew my father's father, but I had a lot of second-hand knowledge of him. He was a banker who lost everything in a financial collapse in the mid-19th century. His son, George – for whom I was named – had to leave the "public" school, Eton, and find work for himself and his family. He found it in the London docks where he went to work as a clerk in an import-export business. He learned the business well, knowing that the only place he could go into that business would be America.

He came here and became a success, specializing in Japanese antique art. He learned to speak and read Japanese and traveled to Japan eleven different times where he was treated with such great respect that he was invited to be the first white man to descend into the crater of Mount Fujiyama. His reputation for integrity was passed on to his son, my father, who passed it on to me. I never knew my grandfather, but he was still alive when my father and mother were getting to know and love each other. My mother had wonderful words for the man who became her father-in-law. After he died, which was before I was born, his widow – my grandmother – built a home in the Eastern Adirondacks and called it Arrochar, named for the Scotland town where young George Hamilton used to spend summers with his family.

I first visited Scotland when I was nineteen and touring Europe. I visited Glasgow and Edinburgh then, but did little else except to promise myself I would come back. My return would take place when I was assigned as a surgeon to an Army hospital in Germany. I traveled the Scottish mainland then and left for home promising I would return. The return would come several years later when I decided to take a voyage of memory to Scotland. I flew to Glasgow, rented a car, and started driving around Western Scotland where I developed a strong sense that it would soon be time for me to go to the Hebrides. I had been attracted to those islands when I was a junior in college, hearing a lovely piece on my roommate's hi-fi that turned out to be Mendelssohn's Hebrides Overture. It called to me.

After I got established in my professional career in Maine, I felt the call to go to the Hebrides. I flew to Glasgow, rented a car there, and started driving west. I found myself in the town of Oban, a ferry terminal for four of the Western Isles. I got a room there, and when I got to the ferry dock the next morning the ferry just landing was making the short trip over to the Isle of Mull. During the crossing, I read what I could find about Mull, which led me to a small island on the western end of Mull, Iona... famous for its religious site, Iona Abbey. I decided to make it part of my journey. I spent several hours becoming acquainted with the rich history of the place. It was a beautiful religious/spiritual experience.

I left Iona in time to get to Tobermorey at the northern end of Mull and a short ferry boat ride over to the mainland. There, I found my way north to the ferry at Mallaig that took me to Armadale on the island of Skye. I had a splendid time driving around that island, heading toward the port town of Uig. The further I got toward Uig, the stronger the sense that I was going home.

I had a B&B reserved in the town of Portree, which is about halfway up the West Coast to Uig. I had a stunning experience there. As I drove into the town. I saw the white "H" on a blue background that got my physician's attention. I decided I would like to see the local hospital; so, I followed the signs to it, and found myself looking at a single-story building with a sizable parking space. As I pulled into a parking spot, a cracker box ambulance pulled in and backed up to an entrance to the hospital. Two men got out and I, a certified trainer in prehospital emergency care, engaged them in brief conversation to see how their emergency service worked. They had come to pick up a very sick man to take him to the large Raigmore Hospital in Inverness, three hours away.

They invited me into the hospital. When I entered, I looked down the corridor to my left and saw the nurse at her station writing... likely the notes needed for the transfer. They pointed to the room where the ill man was to be found. They thought that I might like to see him, considering what I had earlier told them about my reason for visiting the hospital. I stepped quietly into the room and saw a man who was terminally ill probably from an overwhelming septic infection. The shaman in me became aware that his soul was a presence near the body, but not in, the man's body. It was still and at peace. There was nothing more there for me, so I left the hospital and drove to my B&B.

I checked in and was told about a restaurant in the town that served good food. I went there and had a good supper. When I got back to the B&B, I went straight to my room and went to bed. When I got up the next morning, I made ready to leave and went to breakfast. There, I told the woman who owned the B&B about my experience of the day before. Her eyes got big as she said, "That was my grandfather you're talking about. They got him on the road to Inverness. He had a heart attack halfway there. They got him started again and when they drove into the grounds of the hospital in Inverness, he had another heart attack and they couldn't get him going. What you have just told me has made it so much easier for me to accept his death knowing that he was at peace." She continued, saying, "You clearly have a gift, and I'm deeply grateful to you for what you have done for me."

With that gift for both of us, I got on the road to Uig, where a ferry took a long route across open water to the town of Tarbert on the island of Lewis. A fairly long drive northeast took me to Stornoway, the main town of the Western Isles and the capital of Lewis and Harris where I had another B&B room. At breakfast the next morning, the owner said, "You're goin' to the Standin' Stones at Callanish, ain't ya?" I had previously known nothing about them. What she said piqued my curiosity; so, I asked her how to get to see the stones. She gave me the directions and I found my way there. I parked in the visitors parking area that had placards around it describing its history. I paid no attention to them, but felt instead a clear mind to explore the area,

I started clattering around on the granite ledges and green fields amongst all the stones in this "Monumental, megalithic ruins site with a ring of stones

6

surrounding an imposing central monolith." Without a pause in my "clatter" I said aloud, "I've been here before… 6000 years ago."

I soaked up much spiritual energy walking among those old, old stones of a primitive granite called "Lewisian gneiss[ii]." Satisfied (and saturated), it was time to go back to my car and read what was on the plaques. They told me that 6000 years ago was when the people from the East came to this island, found this place, and started building this monument. I had a distinct sense, confirmed by my readings, that the Druids used this area for their practices. I had the sense that this explained a long-standing interest in Druidism and Druids.

I knew that I had received what I had come for, and found my way back to the Scottish mainland, the Glasgow Airport, and my flight home. I knew why I had made this journey… if I may be forgiven for being so bold, it is my sense that Callanais (another name for Callanish) was where my soul came into human life for this journey. I do not know if this incarnation is the last part of my soul's journey. It may be or it may not be.

Healers

I had them on both ancestral sides. I'll start with my father's side because it is older…. my paternal grandmother, Bertha, was raised in a simple Presbyterian family. She married George, the Scot, and had four children by him in the 1880's and 90's. In the first decade of the 20th century, she was attracted to the form of Christian Science that came from Augusta Stetson at the turn of the 20th century. She and her older daughter, Margaret, (my "Aunt Peg") joined the Church of Christ Scientist. Her older son, my father, joined with the two, and their younger brother, Minard, did not. Her younger daughter, Amy Gordon (my "Aunt Gordon"), was born in 1892. When she was 14, she developed severe menstrual blood loss (p. 12).

Her mother's devotion to the beliefs of Augusta Stetson made a visit to a physician impossible. Her Presbyterian father sensed the nature of the problem and took a quiet moment to talk with Amy Gordon about her health condition. She told him, and he responded with, "And the Christian Scientists' prayers aren't helping…" to her "No," he replied, "and they won't let you go

7

to a doctor?" To her affirmative reply, he said, "Let's get you out to Toledo, Ohio, to visit your Aunt Amy Taft... she'll take care of you." Amy Gordon agreed, and they "pulled the wool" over the eyes of the Christian Scientists and got the adolescent girl on the overnight train to Toledo. When she got off the train her Aunt Amy commented on her pale appearance and asked her if she would like to see a doctor. Young Amy's "Yes" got an immediate trip to a surgeon who performed an urgent hysterectomy three days later, saving her life... and setting her on a remarkable professional career.

Amy Gordon knew that she was "barren" and could never marry. She followed an academic interest, went to Bryn Mawr College, where she found a deep interest in social work. She followed that call, winding up as an assistant professor of social work at the New York School of Social Work from 1923 to 1957. She lived in New York with a long-time partner, and I used to visit her often because of her great wisdom and experience. One day, during a visit, I started to explore "God". She interrupted me with, "Toby, I want you to know that the "God" of my mother, your father, and our sister doesn't work for me. Maybe I am an atheist, but there's one thing I know... I love human beings." She was a "giant" in the social work field, and undoubtedly had a great deal to do with my choice of medicine for my professional career. I have a black and white photograph of her, and every time I look up from this computer, I see that picture... and, next to it there are two photos of my lovely wife... no other photos anywhere else in my studio.

Aunt Peg was a Christian Science practitioner who lived in eastern New York state with her partner, Vida, in a lovely old cape in the town of Lewis, just north of the Essex County seat, Elizabethtown. She had an established reputation as a healer that proved itself to me one humid spring day at my home in Short Hills, New Jersey... just the kind of weather that would spread poison ivy and give me itches and blisters on every exposed part of my body. I was getting just such a reaction one day when the telephone rang. Because I was alone in the house, I picked it up, and it was Aunt Peg calling to talk with her brother. She asked me how I was; so, I told her I was "coming down" with poison Ivy. She reminded me of her Christian Science work and asked me if I would like it if she read "the lesson" for me. That was "okay" with me, and I told her so. The itch stopped overnight and the blisters dried up within three days... and I was expecting a week of itchy suffering! After that, I made it a point to call her whenever I was coming down with poison ivy to ask her to read the "lesson" for me. It always worked. Her healing travelled the 300 miles between Short Hills, New Jersey, and Lewis, New York, almost as if the distance never mattered..

My mother was a healer with great healing energy in her hands. She was born into and raised in a doctor's family. Her father was a "General Practitioner" in Lachine, Quebec, a suburb of Montréal. He was much loved and respected by his patients. His reputation as a caring physician led the people of the Kahnawake Mohawk Territory south of the St. Lawrence River across from Lachine to ask him to be their doctor. He was honored by the request and accepted it. He was a graduate of the Faculty of Medicine of McGill University, as was a cousin practicing pediatrics in Mendham, New Jersey, not far from Short Hills where I grew up. I used to visit him to learn more about McGill Medicine. His humanity and reputation led me to obtain my medical education in that medical faculty.

Chapter 2:
The Early years

My birth

As I refused long ago to deny the non-rational aspects of a patient's life, friends told me about my wounded healer nature. I realize now how my soul responded to that recognition. My life's story demonstrates — as everyone's story can — how it is possible to recognize the purpose behind a soul's incarnation. As I look back over my soul's journey, I can identify several important psychical events that led to my own crisis. The saga begins with my birth in 1933 in New York City and goes on to reveal three soul wounds, the eventual healing of which enabled my transition from the life of a general surgeon to that of a shaman.

The story begins before my conception. In late 1932, my mother miscarried an early pregnancy. Her OB did what he could, and she did what she could. When time came for her to go back home, her doctor said, "The best thing for you, Molly, would be to get pregnant right away." She did as her doctor told her and got pregnant right away... I was born the following October 1, 1933. She went into labor on September 29. Twenty-four hours later, without any progress in that labor, now nine months along, the contractions ceased... completely. Another twenty-four hours later, her uterus had displayed no signs of labor; so, her OB recommended a Caesarean section. That is how October 1, 1933 became my birth date.

As the story unfolds with my birth, I must introduce a bit of hearsay from my mother that I have integrated into a memory of my birth. I seem to remember a gentle birth because a caesarean section delivered me from her womb. She told me on several occasions that, according to her obstetrician, I had stopped the labor! She got my attention with that statement and gave me occasion to look outside the box of conventional medical thought, for there is no medical experience with any infant stopping its mother's labor.

In any case, I have a visual recollection of a white room with several people in it, dressed in white. A man with kind eyes has his hands around my chest with his thumbs under my chin, and I see a bright window, through which I see a city. My mother gave me the hearsay of her obstetrician's words, "Molly, he is the strangest boy I have ever delivered. I held him up; he opened his eyes; looked around the room as if he'd been here a hundred times before; put his thumb in his mouth; and fell asleep. I've never before had a child do that." He planted a seed that determined an important quality of our mother-son relationship that endures to this day, twenty-five years after her death.

My imaginary playmate

Over the next five years, while I was learning to evaluate my suburban Long Island world with my physical and emotional senses, I had an imaginary playmate — a teacher named Rookie — who was older and wiser than I, an intimate friend who occupied my dreaming and waking hours. Two things happened during this time that I remember to this day: We were spending, as usual, the summer months with my father's mother, who lived in a lovely house she had built in the Eastern Adirondacks. She took it upon herself to acquaint me with the Bible, and used to read scripture to me every Sunday morning. When the time came for her to read the Garden of Eden legend to me, I had already developed a strong sense that God and love were the same thing. When the reading ended, and, as I was leaving her bedroom, the following came to me: "a loving father would never punish his children like that." What I just heard her read to me was not true.

Abandoned...

Rookie and I shared many exciting and dangerous adventures until shortly after I received my first soul wound at the hands of my mother's sister. We had rented a summer cabin on Great Peconic Bay, Long Island, overlooking a clam flat at low tide where I visited the clammers to find out what they were doing with their funny rakes. One day, I saw a garden rake leaning up against the house, with its tines facing outward. (It caught my attention because my father had told me that leaving a rake like that would be dangerous because of what would happen should I ever step on those tines.) I now heard two voices in my mind: one on each shoulder – the left-shoulder voice said, "Oh look at that rake: you can dig clams with it." On the opposite shoulder, a different voice said, "No you can't, the tines are too short." The encouraging voice won out, and I picked up the rake and climbed down the stairs to the beach, not noticing it was high tide, and the clam flat was not to be seen. Naively, I splashed out into the bay, raking eagerly, but getting no quahogs... only rocks. I continued my pursuit of the elusive bivalves until I was completely underwater. My mother's sister, Aunt Brunie, saw me disappear, and dashed into the water, "dressed in her best summer dress", rescuing me from drowning. For years, I could not remember the rescue, even though my mother told me about it every time I refused to go into water over my knees. I could only recall the fun of pursuing the clams and then having something interrupt me that caused me to look up, seeing the last thing I would remember for 50 years—silver ripples overhead.

There can be little doubt that this episode was profoundly traumatic... I could not, no matter how hard I tried, remember what happened after I looked up and saw ripples in the water over my head. That did not scare me. What scared me was what happened next... trauma that I repressed for about 50 years, when H.O.P.E. Groups started getting interested in in healing "the wounded child". A friend who knew of me and H.O.P.E. Groups where we opened each meeting listening to the Grateful Dead song, *Ripples*, connected me to the work of a New Zealand psychologist, David Groves, Ph.D, in Woburn, Mass. He had sent me a full color brochure advertising a workshop called, "The use of metaphor in healing the wounded child within". There, he told us that the last memory before a trauma was a metaphor, and my last memory was the ripples overhead.

At his invitation I told the workshop about my experience, leading him to ask the ripples about what happened next. I was in a slight trance, and the whole episode came clear out of my repressed memories. I felt a crushing sensation around my chest as if I were grabbed by a terrifying monster. That monster revealed itself to be my aunt as she lifted me out of the water, dripping wet and terrified. She spun me around in midair, grabbed me again, and shouted at me, "Toby, you stupid little boy!" Because I had no memory of this, it had a lasting traumatic disordered pattern of thinking. I developed a habit of finding, WITH great sensitivity, what was "stupid" in the behavior of self and others... PTSD!

Shortly after this traumatic episode, I had a dream in which our archenemies trapped Rookie and me and killed us. Looking at our dead bodies, Rookie said, "I'm leaving you now," to which I responded, "Will you be back?" "I will," he said…. I was reassured but sensing somehow that I was without a spirit-guide and would have to learn by myself until it was time for him to come back to work with me. I managed to get along without him for many years, learning – sometimes very painfully – the great value in knowing the value of having a spirit-guide. It would be some fifty years before I would learn the names of the two directors of life: the secular ego and the spiritual soul.

Again…

I sustained a second soul wound as my hormones were beginning to move me into qualitatively new relationships. During the intervening years, a matriarchy of six wonderfully nurturing women raised me, seemingly aware of my ego's strengths and my soul's purpose. My father, the only other male in my immediate family, and I, shared a quiet, nurturing masculine relationship that balanced the powerful feminine energy. The wound came when a talk between my mother and me turned into an argument. I said something that offended her, to which she responded by asking, "How can you say that if you love me?" My reaction was a deep sense of having been abandoned by my mother. It precipitated a slide into studied ambivalence – a senseless life marked by failing academic grades and meaningless behavior patterns that lasted until I was twenty-one years old. It is a wonder that I survived those years, for so many of my actions bordered on the suicidal. In retrospect, it was a life without apparent purpose, and I was free to cruise through it as I was free to walk the streets of Forest Hills, Long Island, back in the 1930's. Today, someone would have taken me to a psychiatrist who would have labeled this a "depression" and placed me on medication. Had that happened, life might well have taken me elsewhere.

And again…

My third soul wound was a near fatal accident I shall describe in Chapter 3.

It wasn't all thorns: Events can be beneficial; four things happened in my early years that had profound and very beneficial effects on how my life developed.

I remember them well to this day, and I honor and respect them. I shall cover them in the next chapter I call "Waiting".

Chapter 3:
Waiting

I call this chapter, "Waiting" because, in retrospect, I was waiting to be shown what I was to do here when I "grew up" and had a career… of some sorts. While I was "waiting" I did not waste time, in spite of the fact that my father sensed that I had no direction, and complained about it to my mother. She reassured him with, "He'll be all right, Kenny." And that was that. Of course, in her wisdom, she felt it unwise to tell him what that strange woman in Forest Hills had said to her about my destiny. And it was also important that she seldom would repeat those words to me

The 1938 Long Island hurricane

That summer on Great Peconic Bay, Long Island, ended with the famous 1938 hurricane tearing right through the eastern end of the bay where we had rented that cabin. However, I found the hurricane to be "scary", but not terrifying. The day began with wind and rain for several hours before the eye of the hurricane arrived. My wise mother did not like the sudden stillness, so she went outside, saw the approaching eye wall, and knew it meant danger. She came back indoors, told my sister and me we were in danger, and had to leave. She told us that we were going "to Stella's". Stella worked for us as a maid, and her father had a sizable truck farm on a rise and a strong house where Mom was quite sure we would be safe.

We left the cabin just as the eye wall hit and drove fast down the lane to the road. I remember clearly looking out the rear window at the lane just as trees fell across it… scary, yes, but not terrifying. Out on the road, the wind buffeted our car, but Mom drove well and carefully. I remember stopping suddenly… a big tree had fallen across the road, blocking the road completely. Suddenly, four dark figures appeared in the downpour with a couple of crosscut saws. They quickly cut out a length of the tree trunk, and waved us through. The rest of the drive to Stella's passed uneventfully, and we found welcome there… strange timing….

The Move to Short Hills, NJ

Mom went back to our home in Forest Hills, leaving us in Stella's care for what seems was at least a week. When she showed up next, she told us that she and Dad had decided to sell the house in Forest Hills and move to a town in New Jersey where they had bought a house that would be our home. Stella took good care of us until Mom showed up and drove us to that new home in Short Hills. I left behind that one fearful, suppressed memory, and made an adventure out of the move.

It was time to go to school, and my parents enrolled me in first grade at Buxton Country Day School where I would stay through third grade. I made some friends there, but experienced bullying for the first time in my life. I told my parents about it, and we looked at a change of schools. Glenwood public grade school was but one mile from our home, and it was well recommended by our neighbors. I entered fourth grade, and immediately liked the teacher, Mrs. Wycoff. I made friends with several of the boys and girls in the class, and performed well, challenged most by learning cursive handwriting... at Buxton I was taught to print my letters so I had to work to catch up with the others in Glenwood.

Fifth grade went well. The teacher was competent and pleasant (and I do not remember her name). That year was uneventful, and my grades were high, which made learning a pleasure. In retrospect I enjoyed the prospect of moving into Mrs., Birmingham's sixth grade class. She was a middle-aged woman who loved her work. She was kind and encouraging, and I liked her best of all my teachers. I was passionate about learning everything that was available. As the year went on, it was clear that I had four competitors for top grades: Betsy, Gordon, Barbara, and Eugene. There was no animosity among us... only a competitive friendship.

One day, during recess, Mrs. Birmingham asked to speak with me. I agreed, and in her kind and straightforward way she told me that I had a slight edge over the other four and, if I could get my "B" in penmanship up to an "A", I would be the Valedictorian of our sixth-grade graduation. Challenged, I spent hours getting all the letters to cursively flow from one to another. They flowed and I got the "A" and the award, as she had promised.

That test was to have great benefit in the years to come... the lesson was "stubborn persistence"... a trait needed by any person who would become a General Surgeon. Learning to write well is, to me, an important obligation of any physician. I had an experience in second year medical school that deserves space here.... In the summer after that second year in the McGill Faculty of Medicine, I was an "externe" at The Bataan Memorial Methodist Hospital in Albuquerque, New Mexico. I was assigned to a fine General Surgeon, Joseph Garland Riley, M.D, who specialized in plastic surgery. Dr. Riley had perfect cursive handwriting and mine had gotten sloppy. I commented on the quality of his penmanship one day as he was writing an order. His reply: "Ken, you owe it to your colleagues, nurses and patients to write legibly." Period! Thank you, Mrs. Birmingham. Thank you, Doctor Riley.

Middle School and High School

Back then, the first three years after grammar school were known as "Junior High School". My parents decided that the Short Hills Country Day School across the street from the new house we had just bought had a good curriculum for seventh and eighth grades... Reason? Our new next-door neighbor, Edward R. "Bud" Kast, was the headmaster of that school. He was a fine human, a 1943 graduate of Dartmouth College, and past captain of the Dartmouth football team, for whom I have rich memories.

Kast moved on after one year, and Albert Banning took over as headmaster. He also taught mathematics very well. Two other teachers have been in my mind for years, Mlle. Glazier taught French as only the daughter of a French Sorbonne professor can teach French. It was the only language we could speak in her class! She was a petite fiery French woman, and her way of teaching taught me a lot about languages. The history teacher was "Sir" Haines, a stern, demanding teacher who did not stimulate an interest in history. That would have to wait until I was in college....

When it came to choosing a high school, my mother wanted me to go to a private school, but I resisted; so, I enrolled in the Millburn High School and stayed there for two years. The courses that appealed to me were French and Biology. The man who taught French spoke it terribly (I was comparing him to Mademoiselle Glazier). He had leaned French in North Africa where he was stationed in World War II. I got an "A" very easily from him because languages had an extraordinarily strong appeal for me. The biology teacher and I got along very well, and I got good grades from him. After two years at Millburn High School, it was time for me to go on, and Phillips Exeter Academy called me. I applied there and was accepted, I enjoyed mathematics, physics, and German. I did not like history the first time I took it because it was nothing but a list of items. I took it a second time and it became interesting because the teacher taught it as story, which made it appealing.

Of significance in Phillips Exeter was my meeting with Kendall Kent Kane of Dover, Ohio, my roommate in my first year there. (He is gone now, and I want to give you his full name, because of what happened when we met in our rooms at Exeter.) After sharing our names, he said, "I'm going to be a doctor. How about you?" I said, without any forethought, "Me too." Where that came from, I cannot explain... It was simply something I knew from deep inside. My academic performance was very average, and the guidance counselor recommended that I consider going to Haverford College. I remember him saying, "I am quite certain we can get them to accept you." He told me that Haverford was a Quaker college, and I had had an enjoyable experience as a six-year-old reading Marguerite de Angeli's charming book about a willful Quaker girl in pre-Civil War Philadelphia, the title of which was "Thee Hannah". I applied with average grades from Phillips Exeter and was accepted.

I had a sense of just wandering around through educational fields. I did not know why I was there. I learned to smoke cigarettes and to get drunk. I had a bright spot in my life when I was nineteen that gave me a clearer sense of direction. My mother, born a Canadian, remained a Canadian her whole life in spite of the fact that she became a naturalized citizen of the United States during World War II because when she would drive to and from Montréal where her family lived, it was always a challenge at the border where the Canadian woman had two American children.

When Queen Elizabeth II was to experience her coronation on June 2, 1953, my dear mother insisted that I go to England for the coronation and then spend some time touring Europe... by motorcycle. She persuaded my father of the value of the trip, and he accepted. I was to watch the coronation parade at Hyde Park Corner, buy a motorcycle and tour as I wanted, meeting my mother and sister in Zermatt, Switzerland, and climb the Matterhorn with a Swiss guide.

My father, a climate control engineer, had a close friend and colleague who was a Dane. The Dane offered me the opportunity to meet three men of his acquaintance in Copenhagen. One of them was the chief of a medical department in the University of Copenhagen, and meeting him was the last of three important events, each one of which was more important than the actual coronation itself.

The first event was an accident on my motorcycle that was an exquisitely timed experience on a road just north of Rome. I was comfortably touring my way north, when I decided I would like to have a cigarette and I would light it while I was riding my bike. Things did not go well with the lighting procedure and I drifted off the road into a granite Roman milepost that I hit square on. The bike and I vaulted over that heavy piece of granite, separating ever so slightly, landing next to each other, with the bike badly bent, and me completely unhurt! A car stopped and offered me a ride up the road to a town where there was an inn that I could stay in. I accepted the offer, and went to the inn. The son of the inn owner spoke good English, so we arranged for the bike to be picked up and brought to the Inn where I would contact the insurance company to get it fixed.

The following morning, the son of the owner asked me if I would like to go for a ride with him in a new Alfa Romeo convertible owned and driven by a friend of his. I accepted that invitation, and shortly after that his friend showed up with a passenger in the four–passenger Alfa, and the two of us from the inn got in the back seat. It was a beautiful sunny day, and the driver was driving quickly and well. It was a pleasant trip until we crested a steep hill with a farm on either side and a cow crossing the road immediately in front of us – totally unavoidable! But in that instant, we were suddenly on the other side of the cow, never having had that collision! The driver was hard on the brakes, and, when we had stopped, we all looked back, and she was plodding along on the other side of the road as if nothing had ever happened. We all agreed that we had seen something impossible! We continued back to the inn, filled with wonder, accepting the reality of the situation.

I took care of the matter of getting the bike back to England to the BSA people for repair and I got on a train to meet my mother, my sister, and her boyfriend, Alan W, in Zermatt, Switzerland. They had arranged for a climb up the Matterhorn the next day with a family of well-known guides. I was in terrible shape but my guide was very understanding and I made it up the Matterhorn with my sister and her boyfriend. This was exciting. It was a rich experience, and a great thing to know that I had been able to make the climb up and back down again.

We parted ways then, and I went on to Copenhagen. I met with the three men for whom I had introductory letters, and the meeting with the third, the professor of medicine at the University of Copenhagen, was an important part of my life. We had a pleasant meeting, and one of his residents then took me on a tour of this beautiful Danish hospital of white walls and teak fittings. I told the professor that I would very much appreciate the opportunity to do a summer in his hospital as I was going through my McGill education. He said that would be fine, and I would have to get a working knowledge of Danish and three years of medical school behind me. We shook on that and said our goodbyes.

The energy of the Haverford campus was soft and nurturing. Haverford put up with me, however, even though my behavior could have been described as one of being chronically depressed. I thought I would like to major in philosophy, but the professors of that department would not accept me. I asked the professors of German if they would accept me as a major, and they agreed. My performance in their classes was, to put it succinctly, mediocre. I was to fail my first attempt at writing my senior comprehensive exam, but something else had happened in November of my senior year. I *knew* I was to become a M.D, helped by my first meeting with Ken Kane in 1941 (p. 36). I also knew that I was to graduate from the Faculty of Medicine of McGill University in Montréal where my mother's father and one of her cousins had received their medical education. It was more than a decision; it was a "knowing."

I told my father that I wanted to go to McGill, and I needed an interview with the Dean. His reaction was favorable. He told me that a legacy from his Uncle Norman would pay the McGill tuition and he would pay my airfare to Montréal and back, staying there with my mother's sister, Brunie... the same Brunie who had shouted at me for being a stupid little boy when I was about five years old trying to dig clams on a rocky bottom at high tide with a garden rake!

As I was moving into a disastrous senior year in college, I *knew* that I would need to I commit myself to doing whatever was needed to get into medical school. The only school I had in mind was the Faculty of Medicine at McGill University in Montreal, Canada. I wrote the Dean, got an appointment with him, and my father gave me the round-trip airfare ticket to Montreal.

I had a simple flight to Montréal, spent the night with my aunt, and went to the Dean's office at McGill the next day. He asked to see my transcript. When I gave it to him, he took one look and said, "I can't accept you with this transcript."

My reply... "I know that, but I want to be a McGill graduate; so please tell me what I must do in order for you to accept me."

His immediate answer... "You're clearly an intelligent young man, but you're going to have to prove it to me. You must also show me that you're capable of doing the work that a physician has to be able to provide. I'm going to ask you to take a full postgraduate year at an approved college or university, taking four courses in premedical science in each of two semesters – no botany, mind you – and I must ask you to get straight A's. Wait a minute... I want you to take organic chemistry over again and I'll let you have a 'B' in it but that's the only one. Is that clear?" I said it was.

He then said, "You may want to go into the Army for two years to grow up. In any case you will still have to take that post-graduate year of pre-medical courses, if you want me to accept you." I knew I would have to sleep on that one, but the basic terms of the agreement were completely acceptable to me. We shook hands on it, and I flew home...

That flight home was remarkable... something happened that deeply appealed to the mystic in me: flying out of Montréal, the plane went through a thin overcast, and from my right-hand side seat, I could see in the next cloud layer yet above and to the west was a perfectly round hole in the cloud and the sun was behind it off to one side, illuminating the entire hole with gold. I knew that I had made a perfect set of choices.

23

When I got home, I told my father about the agreement, pleasing him to no end. He said that his Uncle Norman had left me a legacy that would likely cover my McGill tuition. He suggested that I go to Rutgers University, Newark, New Jersey, and commute from home to save room and board. He introduced me to Dean Phelan at Rutgers, whom he knew and respected highly. It was but a 20-minute train ride from Short Hills to Newark, and a five-minute walk from there to the University. I told Dean Phelan what I needed and he accepted me unconditionally as a graduate student. I signed up for four courses in each of two semesters, and gave the Dean at McGill eight A's. I took my senior comps in German that spring, and passed them. It was perfectly clear to me that I was literally marking time until it was right for me to go to medical school and become a physician.

All this delighted my mother. She had been gently steering me towards Medicine for many years. I was now happy and at peace with myself. I knew that I was doing what I had come to earth to do. The waiting was over.

Chapter 4:
Ego meets Soul

Ego

My ego did not set up the introduction to the Grateful Dead song, *Ripple*, whose funky, country-western tune I heard first on my car radio in the spring of 1987. I was driving, paying attention to the road, when that tune caught my attention. I gave the words no thought, and, at the end of the piece, when the DJ mentioned the name of the song, which I did not get, he also said, "by the Grateful Dead," and I got that! I set an intention to find that piece, and by a set of circumstances that could be called "luck", I went to a music store and chose *one* of the two different "Best Of" cassettes in the Grateful Dead display section. I knew that *it* had to contain that nameless song. Later that evening I played the tape, and there it was… *Ripple.* I put the tape aside, playing it for the second time a few weeks later as background music while driving with a friend of mine to do some spring high water river running in solo canoes. At the end of our run, he stayed behind with friends, so I drove home alone. When I got out on the open road, I felt like listening to *Ripple.* I started the tape, and, to my astonishment and delight, *Ripple was perfectly queued up,* and the opening words sang to my soul: "If my words did glow with the gold of sunshine, and my tune were played on the harp unstrung, would you hear my voice come through the music? Would you hold it near; as it were your own?"

My ego did not set up the circumstances that led me to take part in the Elisabeth Kübler-Ross five-day intensive called *Life, Death, and Transition.* Here, several important things happened to me: first, I was overwhelmed by the stories of sexual abuse that many of the participants told and to which I responded with deep grief. Second, I had a mystical experience with my long-dead parents. My weeping woke me at dawn on the third day, and I wandered out into a foggy, light drizzle, listening to that Grateful Dead song, *Ripple.* I played it repeatedly as I wandered down a lovely maple-lined lane. Suddenly, I saw my long dead parents, my mother first, fully dressed, sitting in a simple living room chair, looking at me with her yellow-brown eyes. I thanked her for waiting for me. I told her that I loved her, and that she was "free to go". She smiled a beautiful smile and vanished into the fog.

I sensed a presence in the mist near me. It was a charcoal outline of my father in front of a similar outline that I sensed was his father. I said, "I love you and I've always loved you. Thank you for waiting. You're free to go." As I said those words, I saw a black cord extend from my heart through his into his father's heart. As I watched, it began to glow, faintly red at first, then brighter and brighter to yellow-white when it burst into flame, freeing the two images to disappear into the mist.

These two acts of graceful forgiveness brought my grief to an end, and I moved into a state of deep, deep peace. In that moment, I had a clear sense that both had been sexually abused. Later, as the story telling resumed, and more tales of sexual abuse came forth, I stayed at peace. The grieving was indeed over. That evening, I told the group of 85 people what had happened to me that morning. The facilitator who was with me said, "Elizabeth calls that 'Divine Intervention,'" to which I agreed. My life changed after that, and I knew that my ego had nothing to do with creating the events that led to the transformation. I also knew that I felt a great deal better about me and that I had let go of about 95 percent of my old anger.

My mother's hurtful question about my ability to love (p. 32) teamed up with my introverted, feeling nature, and I lost my sense of self-worth. I slid into a state that took me from being top of my class in grade school to the bottom of my class in college. It was a process that took ten years to complete. Halfway through it, though, I somehow knew with crystal clarity that the only profession for me was medicine. It certainly had a lot to do with the fact that my father, his mother, and his older sister were Christian Scientists. And my mother came from a family of physicians. I know that sounds crazy, but that is how my family was. So how much of this intention was a product of my genes, my nature, and my environment; my nurture, cannot be clearly established. When I couple all that with a passion to fix things, a pair of good hands, and a high mechanical attitude, I had to become a surgeon.

In spite of the fact that I was born into a spiritual, healing, Christian Science, Episcopal, medical family, in this dark time I could not turn to the God of their understanding for help. I had lost the way. Help came from another avenue, my father's younger sister, Amy Gordon Hamilton, called by all, "Gordon". Aunt Gordon had nearly died from severe menstrual hemorrhage when she was fourteen years old. Her elder brother (my father), her older sister, and their mother tried to get God to stop the bleeding with Christian Science healing prayer. It did not help. Gordon's own Aunt Amy, for whom she was named, lived hundreds of miles away in Toledo, Ohio. My grandfather intuited all that was going on and suggested to Amy Gordon that she go to Toledo to her namesake Aunt Amy Taft, having told his sister-in-law about the young woman's plight, and the older woman arranged for Gordon to come to Toledo. On her arrival in Toledo, her aunt Amy saw how ill she was, and they went straightaway to a doctor who performed the life-saving hysterectomy three days later[iii].

When I was in my young adult years, Aunt Gordon and I used to talk about many things. She was a well-educated woman who had become an assistant-dean of the New York School of Social Casework at Columbia University. In the male-dominated professions of the thirties and forties, she chose to use her middle name, Gordon, over her first name, Amy. Her pen name became "A. Gordon Hamilton," and more than once, when she was introduced to a person familiar with her work, that person would exclaim, "You're Gordon Hamilton? I thought you were a man!"

Our minds worked in similar ways, and I loved being with her. Once, when I brought up the subject of God, she said to me, "Toby, you know my story, and you know that the prayers of my mother, sister, and brother didn't work for me, but surgery did. Because of that, I don't know about what they call God. I guess I am an atheist... but I love human beings."

As far as I was concerned, Gordon helped free me from any magical beliefs that the God of my childhood would always take care of me in the way in which little Toby wanted. I saw that if anyone were to direct my life it would have to be me. In my mind, I had become a single human being whose existence was purely a chance interaction of atoms and molecules. I had come from dust and I would fade away into dust when I died, so it was up to *me* to do what I wanted to do in life. I took charge of my life and assumed full responsibility for creating my disastrous college experience. I assumed full responsibility for becoming a physician, flew to Montreal and negotiated the terms under which the Dean at McGill would accept me into that famous medical school (detailed on p. 65).

In retrospect, Gordon had made a spiritual statement when she said, "I love human beings." In her relationship *with humans*, she had a clear sense that there was a fundamental presence behind all existence. She had a remarkable wisdom and peacefulness that I remember clearly and well. Her caring and wisdom saved her life on more than one occasion when a distraught person showed up in her office with a gun, intending to kill her for threatening behavior. Aunt Gordon lived in the here-and-now press of New York City for most of her adult life. She always saw the greatness and wonders of humanity, and I gained greatly. Through her, I came to see atheism as a spiritual ally, because it challenged the existence of a judging, condemning God. In the years since then, I have plumbed the depths of most of the great religions. I have learned that spirituality, whether you call it theism and atheism all come down to the same thing... there is a single, compassionate, non-judgmental, Uncaused Cause from which all things spring.

Soul

Every life is the journey of a soul, rich in divine purpose. A soul incarnates to bring its spiritual wisdom into a specific encounter with a finite, secular ego, creating thereby a unique experience of life. This experience comprises a mythic saga—a hero's shamanic journey through grave crises of pain and joy, shadow and light. It becomes a single volume in the encyclopedia of that soul's journey to God—a journey without distance to a goal that never changes[iv]. The finished encyclopedia of experience is a soul's sacred gift to God in return for God's original gift of life. To help a human being discover the soul's purpose brings meaning, value, and purpose to the chaos of an ego-directed life... and allows old wounds to heal.

The works of Mircea Eliade[v] and Michael Harner[vi] helped introduce the soul-centered way of the shaman to our Western consciousness. They describe a worldwide distribution of shamanic ritual practices that assist in healing soul wounds. Shamans believe that our essence – the soul – is tender and shy, chipping under the strain of mild traumas such as a sprained ankle or shattering under the duress of a violent attack. Shamans recover these fragments and reintegrate them into the wounded soul. Shamans come from a cohort of "wounded healers," all of whom have specific repetitive patterns of dysfunctional behaviors through which they seek to heal their own soul wounds and, in turn, the wounds of the wounder. When the soul wounds heal, this behavior ends and the shaman emerges from their disease as the butterfly emerges from its chrysalis, with pain and struggle that it must endure alone, for any attempt to help it kills it. The result, like the butterfly, is a thing of beauty.

In contemporary Western society, this creates a medical conundrum—how to recognize a hero's journey and not interfere with it in the face of years of training that focus on disease as something "wrong" rather than as part of a soul's journey. The answer lies in recognizing the soul's presence in illness and providing the specific help it asks for. We cannot reduce this work to an algorithm, for it requires listening to an individual's life story with body, mind, and soul; identifying the mythic saga in it; asking the soul to describe its purpose; and then meeting its needs for technical help. The task requires patience and compassion, the fruits of which are immeasurable. Meeting the needs of the soul returns art to the practice of medicine and heals *its* soul wounds... wounds that come from making life a rational, scientifically understood phenomenon.

As I refused long ago to deny the non-rational aspects of a patient's life, friends told me about my wounded healer nature. I realize now how my soul responded to that recognition. My life's story demonstrates—as everyone's story can—how it is possible to recognize the purpose behind a soul's incarnation. As I look back over my soul's journey, I can identify several important psychical events that led to my own crisis. The saga begins with my birth in 1933 in New York City that I described in Chapter 2 and goes on to reveal three soul wounds, the eventual healing of which enabled my transition from the life of a general surgeon to that of a shaman.

Over the next five years, while I was learning to evaluate my suburban Long Island world with my physical and emotional senses, I had an imaginary playmate—a teacher named Rookie—who was older and wiser than I was... an intimate friend who occupied my dreaming and waking hours. Two things happened during this time that I remember to this day: in the summer of my third or fourth year, we were spending, as usual, the summer months with my father's mother, who lived in a lovely house she had built in the Eastern Adirondacks. She took it upon herself to acquaint me with the Bible and used to read scripture to me every Sunday morning. When the time came for her to read the Garden of Eden legend to me, I already had a strong sense that God and love were the same thing. When the reading ended, and, as I was leaving her bedroom, the following came to me: "a loving father would never punish his children like that. What I just heard her tell me was not true."

Abandoned...

Rookie and I shared many exciting and dangerous adventures until shortly after I received my first soul wound at the hands of my mother's sister when she rescued me from drowning (p. 30)

Shortly after this episode, I had a dream in which our archenemies trapped Rookie and me and killed us. Looking at our dead bodies, Rookie said, "I'm leaving you now," to which I responded, "Will you be back?"

"I will," he said…. I had just lost a soul friend[vii].

I managed to get along without him for many years, learning—sometimes very painfully—how to rely on my ego's resources. I sustained my second soul wound as my hormones were beginning to move me into qualitatively new relationships. During the intervening years, a matriarchy of six wonderfully nurturing women raised me, seemingly aware of my ego's strengths and my soul's purpose. My father – the only other male in my family – shared a quiet, nurturing masculine relationship that partially balanced the powerful feminine energy.

The soul wound when I was eleven led me to an enduring perception of my mother abandoning me (p.32). It gradually healed with the love flowing from these wonderful women, and both of my parents. As a result, I came to feel that this experience was not my soul's purpose when it incarnated. However, my sense is that this was essential to the development of my spiritual nature – that nature of having a divine assignment given very early – even before birth. Through the forces that have directed my life, I have learned to recognize the signs of soul wounds in my family. Suffering from perceptions of abandonment, my soul kept to the background except for the occasions when it needed to steer my car or my footsteps away from certain death. It emerged with power in the autumn of my senior year in college, not long after my twenty-first birthday. It gave me a strong hint of its purpose, aware that this hint would give my life purpose, direction, and meaning[viii].

I came to know through the benefits of the healing presences in my family that I was to develop a career in medicine. Developing that career choice was challenging and rewarding. The 1953 agreement I had made with the Chief of the Department of Medicine in the Royal Hospital of Copenhagen held influential promise that was far greater than what I ever imagined. It led to the choice to become a McGill physician. When McGill accepted me, I got along well with my studies there. The summer externeship after my third year at McGill was possible because I had earlier met the requirements to study at that Danish hospital. However, within two weeks of my arrival I met the woman I have been married to for over 40 years, so I did not learn much medicine. Long ago, we reached a clear understanding that my real purpose in going to Denmark was not to study medicine but to meet her.

I graduated from McGill with honors in several subjects, married my Danish sweetheart, and performed resident duties well, ending with a four-year general surgical residency in Iowa City, Iowa. As a McGill medical student and to avoid being drafted for general medical work, I had obligated myself to volunteer to serve in the military as a general surgeon. I wanted a European assignment to be close to my wife's Danish family and to my aging parents living in Spain. With this purpose in mind, I went to the Office of the Surgeon General of the Army and convinced the interviewing officer that my fluency in French, Danish, and German and an established acceptance by people of those countries would make me a good ambassador. The army assigned me to Germany where we lived off base, learning to speak German and learning German customs. There, I discovered the art and beauty of motorless flight. Thus, I set the stage for my third soul wound, a wound that contained three important parts of the life of the shaman: the descent into the underworld with a near-death experience, a ritual dismemberment, and a return to life transfigured.

After my obligation to Uncle Sam ended, my family and I returned to eastern New York to a house that a favorite aunt had willed to us. To make ends meet while I sought a position as a general surgeon, I worked as an emergency room physician in the small local hospital. There I read an advertisement for a general surgeon to fill a position in a rural Maine town and clearly remembered the description of climate and geography that my wife and I had created five years earlier on a sultry August day in Iowa. Our complaints about that environment led us to daydream of a cool rural town with hills, trees, and four seasons — all within an hour of the ocean. I looked in a road atlas and saw that this Maine town was forty miles from the ocean, had a population of 12,000, and nestled in the foothills of the White Mountains. I submitted my résumé and the hospital promptly responded with an invitation to meet with its staff and administration. On our arrival, we became aware that we had earlier described the region with remarkable precision... it felt as if we were coming home. We have lived there ever since. The intention – a chosen course of action – we created in Iowa manifested with the help of frequent discussions in Germany. By now, I was becoming aware that the purposes of my life seemed to come from a source far beyond me. Furthermore, with my wife choosing to share in them, they became even more powerful.

Chapter 5:
Metamorphosis

Introducing the chapter:

"Metamorphosis" comes from a Greek word that means "transform". The Encyclopedia Britannica defines it as: "a: change of physical form, structure, or substance especially by supernatural means; b: a striking alteration in appearance, character, or circumstances." It is a word that is commonly associated with the process that creates a butterfly. Its egg turns into a caterpillar, that becomes a chrysalis with a hard shell in which the digestive juices in the caterpillar dissolve itself, leaving its central nervous system intact. Specialized "imaginal disks" with a different DNA start to multiply and build the adult butterfly. In the case of the Monarch butterfly, that adult living anywhere in North America knows how to fly to its winter home in Mexico. Whereas it takes only one generation of Monarchs to get to Mexico, it takes several generations to get to its spring/summer home to the North.

My work with H.O.P.E. helps people to completely restructure the way they see themselves and others. This is not a physical change so much as it is a psycho-spiritual change. I have learned to see this change in a person's appearance yes, the expressions of anger and fear are clearly recognizable whenever they're present. The shift to peace is also clearly recognizable. I deeply appreciate seeing this metamorphosis appear. I shall now describe for you my experience with my own metamorphosis.

My Crash

As a well-trained country surgeon who had graduated from a program that specialized in training country surgeons, I took on more than I could handle alone and entered into a terrible spiral of overwork. One lovely August 1972 afternoon, exhausted from saying "Yes" too many times, I had become embittered, resentful, and pessimistic. I sought peace in flying a beautiful glider that I had brought back from Germany in 1970 I went for a glider flight that ended in a near-fatal crash. I was setting up to land at an unfamiliar airfield near Augusta, Maine's capital city, when a gust of wind broke up my landing pattern. In my state of mind, I overreacted and put the plane in a stall a few hundred feet above the earth. In the face of developing a fatal "spin" that would have landed me on my head, I remembered the words I heard in Germany where I learned to fly gliders... from a WWII Messerschmidt fighter pilot. On takeoff, he had lost control of his glider and recovered in time to put the controls in the right place to prevent a fatal spin. He told me and another pilot what he had been taught to do if he lost control of the ailerons in his Messerschmidt.

This was a life-saving gift five years later... instead of crashing headfirst and dying, I positioned the glider so that it drove a wing tip into the ground, and the crumpling of that whole wing lessened the energy of the crash so that the stump of what had been the wing caused a cartwheel that I would survive at the cost of a broken ankle and three vertebrae. The result... thirteen days in the hospital with my broken bones... and the awareness that I had brought on the accident myself. It was a wakeup call to deal with a family anger issue that would take the next fifteen years to resolve through a variety of life situations, the next coming in 1975

As the glider was about to hit the ground, I sensed that I could die... and I was incredibly calm, wondering if the dying would hurt. The crash knocked me out, and when I recovered my senses, my various broken bones caused pain that was tolerable until a physician – a fellow "priest," (if you will) – in the local emergency room refused me pain medication pending the arrival of the orthopedic surgeon – a "high priest" – who would take care of my fractures and pain. Abandoned by a member of my own "priesthood", I plunged into a rocky descent into the underworld; my pain became a torture over which I had no control. The first action of the high priest was to restore comfort to my broken body with a "magical potion"—an intravenous narcotic.

My spiritual descent deepened; the surgeon told me I needed surgery to treat the injury to my foot – a ritual dismemberment. The next stage of the descent into the underworld contained more magical potion—a general anesthetic that overwhelmed me with terrifying blackness. For the next three hours, the high priest disassembled my smashed right ankle, removing all semblance of a joint between my leg and my foot. He reassembled it with the proper ritual of closing the wounds and encasing the leg in white plaster of Paris.

The transfiguration was, however, incomplete. When the high priest changed the plaster cast just before my discharge, he appeared dissatisfied with the alignment of my foot and leg. He twisted my foot inward, just enough to create a permanent deformity that would increase my physical limitations. The presence of a white plaster cast that went from my toes to my groin signaled the completion of the dismemberment and transfiguration. I would wear several more casts over the next four months while the transfiguration solidified. My body healed, but my soul had suffered a third wound.... It would yet heal.

In 1975, in a crisis of anger and anxiety, I found a practice that helped me relieve the feelings that had nearly killed me. I did not yet know that all of this rage and dread was a part of my story with a greater purpose. A new "high priest"– the businessperson Earl Nightingale[ix] – came into my life just when I needed him. Earl's purpose in life was to teach the historical aspects of achieving success – the progressive realization of a worthy ideal – by remembering and developing the purpose of a life, thereby effecting a powerful shift in attitude.

I introduced Nightingale's principles to my patients, who found them wonderfully helpful in their recovery from my operations and their illnesses; with their encouragement, I sought a greater experience with psychology. I met a gifted psychiatrist who had survived a hero's journey and through him, I was able to acknowledge my soul wounds. A year later, with the skillful help of a psychologist with a shamanic nature, I recovered the soul fragment that had stayed behind in the waters of Great Peconic Bay because of the clam-digging trauma. He took me back to the trauma and through it; he let me experience the terrifying sensation of someone grabbing me from behind, lifting me out of the water, and screaming at me for being stupid. This soul recovery evoked a great sense of peaceful relief. With it, a dysfunctional behavior of stupidity that had inexorably repeated itself every four years ended completely, transformed into a shamanic ability to help others heal their wounds.

The next part of my soul recovery – a profound spiritual experience – and related to my second soul wound, took place at an intensive workshop in a Shaker village fifty-five miles from my home. There, I experienced profound grief for unknown reasons. After two nights with little sleep, I found myself wandering around the foggy village just before dawn, listening to the Grateful Dead song, *Ripple,* an exquisite hymn of hope and meaning. Through eyes dimmed by tears and fog, I saw both of my long-dead parents hovering in the mist. I was able to say, "I love you both and I have always loved you. Thank you for waiting. You're free to go." Love flowed between us and they disappeared into the mist. That intention of the fifteen-year-old to find out about love had been realized.

I felt relief penetrate deep into my core, which led the next day to an experience of divine power. In preparation for a karaoke of *Ripple* in that evening's closing ceremony, I sang and danced it repeatedly, entering a rapture that led me down the lane to the Shaker cemetery with the purpose of sharing it with the Shaker souls whose hymn, Simple Gifts, described their practice of entering rapture. Standing in front of the latched cemetery gate and surrounded by maple trees in brilliant autumn color, I saw a spirit face in every leaf and asked if I could enter and share the song and my dance. They smiled, and as I reached for the latch, the gate opened well before my hand touched it. Knowing that I had looked into the face of The Mystery and finding myself welcome there, I sang and danced in Its Presence... transformed.

A few weeks later, with peace in my soul, I went to a conference on hospice work where I attended a workshop on forgiveness. I realized then that I had forgiven my parents and myself all the suffering we had shared. In a closing guided imagery, the imaginary companion of my childhood appeared, now younger than I, but the Rookie I had always known. I welcomed him with an open heart.

Shortly after this workshop, I had a dream in which Rookie and I were in a dangerous situation—a hurricane-like tempest that I associated with the incident where we had both lost our lives so many years before. This time, however, Rookie and I escaped the danger. In the peace of the storm's aftermath, we found ourselves in a green field studded with diamonds. Somehow, I knew we were supposed to be there. I asked Rookie if this was the right place, to which he replied, "Yes". I took a large scalpel out of a sheath at my belt and made an incision in the Earth. I reached into the incision and delivered a beautiful, brown-skinned woman who stood on the Earth, hands open towards me, smiling in her gratitude. I knew who she was... the Black Madonna—the Earth Mother. My soul was at peace.

This new life had come to be through me... through the recovery of my soul fragments. With the delivery of this sacred feminine presence, my life assumed a new, higher level of complexity. I had integrated the experience of my ego and soul into one deeper, richer, individual purpose: to help others heal their own souls, as once a shaman helped me heal mine. Now I knew what it meant to die to one's Self. The deeper purpose of my life arose from an alignment of purposes that had taken me on a journey through joy and suffering to the edge of my life. I have returned from the edge to serve a purpose far greater than my ego could ever have imagined and my ego has agreed to commit his strengths to my soul's purpose. My life is now a vital part of the story of my soul's journey: one volume in a sacred encyclopedia of experience that comprises a gift to God in gratitude for God's original gift of Life.

It would be years before I came to see this kind of patient-doctor dialog as soul-talk. But then, again, in 1971 no one was talking about soul. I only knew that when I was present to my patients, I could ask simple personal questions about their lives and their interests and they would tell me. This is a professional *intimacy* that benefited the patient in terms of postoperative comfort and length of stay. They also seemed to need significantly less pain medication than average. They got on their feet sooner, and they start talking about going home after remarkably brief hospital stays... and all of this before the days of *managed* care. *Listening* to my patients told them that I *cared*. This leads me to consider whether it is more important today to *manage* care or to simply care.

My patients taught me that listening to their thoughts and feelings was better than giving advice about their lives. They accepted *clinical* advice as appropriate to pre-operative counseling, pain management, and discharge instructions, those things in which I had received special education. Listening to them tell me about themselves gave me the power to reflect on their strengths and their gifts, which was not "giving advice" or making a prognosis. They taught me that my reflections were gifts to them that brought us together in a shared focus on their healing and health, from which we both benefited. Some of these people began to tell me that my questions and reflections had helped them to change their lives, and over time, I came to see the depth and richness of this dialog.

Over this same time, I learned from these fine people the kind of questions that were important in helping them effect those changes, and I was able to develop a focus that continually improved my time management. This was important, not because an insurance company was looking over my shoulder, but because there were people in waiting room. I did not over-book or double-book my patients, but I could never predict when a series of words, usually in the form of questions, would spring from the patient's mouth, demanding attention and response. Though I may not have wanted to spend the time listening, the person was telling me s-he needed the time. It was not something to reschedule or prescribe a pill for. The wonderful women who worked for me in my office always knew when this situation arose, and they helped the waiting ones adjust to the situation to everyone's benefit.

Recovery

It took me four months to physically recover to the point where I could operate again. I had been up to full steam for three months when my surgical partner died in a house fire! Suddenly, I was left to cover the general and gynecological surgical needs of the hospital... alone. Would I be able to take on those responsibilities in view of my mistakes in the preceding year?

While all of us at the hospital reeled from that blow, I found I was able to perform my duties well because I had learned important lessons in that accident. I did not have to deny the feelings of loss and grief, but I could give myself time for them in appropriate settings that did not impair my ability to serve. I could pace myself and say "no" when I had to and make appropriate referrals as needed. I could take a day off, having arranged with surgeons in other hospitals to cover our emergencies. This situation made me ever so much more aware of my limitations. It made me promise to myself that I would do my best to avoid repeating the circumstances that had nearly killed me.

I helped the hospital recruit physicians, including a good surgeon just out of his residency, and things looked up... ROSES... with but one big thorn, the anger that had almost killed me in 1972 started coming back, for much the same reason! By 1975, with five new physicians on staff, there were pressures on my time that took me back to the months before my accident, and I found myself becoming extremely anxious with this situation. I thought I had the situation "under control", but it seemed that everyone was angry with me. I complained of this to my practice manager, and he responded by giving me an *INSIGHT* audiotape, produced by Earl Nightingale. He said, as he handed it to me, "Ken, there's a piece on this tape that may help you with that anger feeling." That "piece" was Earl, speaking in his resonant baritone voice, and describing what he called "the law of correspondence". This law, according to Earl, was a variation on the eternal law of "What you sow you reap", namely: "the world always reflects your prevailing attitude back at you." Earl went on to mention that we always *choose* our attitudes, although we might not remember why we made that choice in the first place. The freedom to choose an attitude makes it possible, though not necessarily easy, to change that attitude.[x] Nightingale was fond of saying, "I may not be able to change my mind, but I can change my attitude. Give me about five minutes."[xi] I came to agree with him long before Daniel Goleman's book, *Emotional Intelligence* (Bantam, 2005), was published.

If Nightingale was right, then the anger I saw around me was *mine*. It was extremely painful to admit that he was right, but I knew he was. I now had but one problem, choosing the attitude to replace the anger. I knew that nature abhors a vacuum, and that simply pushing the anger away would result in its immediate, rampaging return. I knew I *had* to work on this, and I had a good place for it... at the stop sign at the first intersection on my way home. For the preceding three months, without fail, I would have to wait for traffic to pass the intersection before I could turn and follow it, for it was always going in my direction. The intersection was *never* clear of traffic—even at two a.m.—and this in a town of only twelve thousand souls!

And almost any day toward dusk, the line of traffic at the stop sign would be long, up to twenty cars long. When this happened, the driver at the head of the cortege had to be a certain old man who lived three miles north of town, and who never drove more than fifteen miles an hour! Imagine my furious anger every time I met him there. Try as I might otherwise, I managed to meet him there two or three times a week!

The afternoon after I first listened to that Nightingale tape, I committed myself to getting to the stop sign without anger, and I found myself saying, "Take it easy." When I got up to leave my office however, I felt anxious. I paused, giving myself permission to identify this feeling for the first time in many years. I found myself saying, "Let it go, Ken. Take it easy." To my surprise, the anxieties settled down—but they returned as soon as I approached my car.

"Let it go, Ken!"

I opened the car door... more anxiety!

"Let it go, Ken! You don't need it! It's not doing you or anyone else any good! Let it go!"

After what still seems like a dozen more of these interactions and affirmations, I got the car started and out on the street. I crawled the one hundred yards to that stop sign, anxiety mounting, and repeating my encouraging words like a mantra. I screwed my eyes up tight so that the only thing I could see was the stop sign. I stopped at it and waited, scared and apprehensive, not really knowing what I was afraid of. It took a major act of will to open them. When I finally did, there was only one car in sight, and I was sitting in it! The relief was so profound that I nearly cried, and I knew that my fear and apprehension had been over the possibility that there would be no traffic at the stop sign. The feeling of relief immediately became an overwhelming feeling of joy.

Though the traffic at the stop sign did not go away forever, there were now plenty of times when the road would be clear when I got to the intersection. Strangest of all though, I never met the old man at the stop sign again. Later, on hearing the expression "when the pupil is ready, the teacher appears," I knew exactly what it meant. That old man had been one of my greatest teachers, although I never knew his name. Several years later, when I told that story at a conference in Florida, a woman came up to me later and told me that she knew that I was talking about her grandfather.

This was a remarkable example of synchronicity or non-coincidental coincidence. It boggled my mind to be aware that I had never met the old man at that intersection prior to three months earlier, and then, after I had chosen to be peaceful inside, I never encountered him there again. I know he drove for several more years because I would occasionally encounter him and his cortege going the opposite way – but never my way.

A new psychology

This was an opening to Earl Nightingale's vast experience with a practical human psychology, the psychology of success. I was encouraged to begin a steady practice of learning more from him and the others associated with his organization, such well-known people as: Brian Tracy, Wayne Dyer, Dennis Waitley, Tom Peters, and Zig Ziglar.[xii] These people were all talking about success and how to achieve it. Nightingale and his friends made the point perfectly clear that there was an historically proven psychology of success that had practical value for the life of every human being. Earl had devoted his lifetime to studying and learning what he later titled *The Essence of Success*[xiii]. It began in 1933 when he was a *twelve-year-old* facing family break-up and poverty in the midst of the Great Depression. At this time, he knew that he had a passion to become a successful businessman. With the help of his local librarian, he began a two-hour daily study of the lives and writings of successful people that he would maintain for the rest of his life.

To Earl and his friends, success was attainable through the limitless resources of the mind, made available by the choice of appropriate attitudes, which resulted in desirable, creative actions. Success was a process, a path, available to everyone who chooses it, and promising relief from the harmful effects of stress. Nightingale defined it as "the progressive realization of a worthy ideal" He went on to say that we are all born with one and the greatest service we can do for self and others is to remember that "worthy ideal" and serve it.

I shared Earl's experience with my patients during these times of listening that I described above. It also seemed that every time Earl, in one of his monthly INSIGHT tapes, helped me make a new discovery in this field, one of the people I was working for was also looking for what I just learned. I found out how to coach these people into choosing different attitudes. I also saw that anger and fear were intimately related, and that neither led to creating a lasting success of anything at all. I saw, instead, that hope and peacefulness gave them the *potential* to direct their lives into more satisfying and meaningful pattern. I was able to encourage them to realize that potential. I discovered the means by which I could effect some of these positive changes during the course of a short office or hospital visit. The experience of circling your soul, as I described in Part Two of my 2002 book, *Soul Circling*, will give you the opportunity to experience such changes for yourself.

After ten years of study and application of these ideas, I sought more training in counseling, and was led to a gifted psychiatrist who taught me a psychology based on attitudes that were fundamental to *how a person moves in relationships.* These moves were: against (anger), away from (fear) and toward (love).[xiv] After we had worked together for nearly two years, this wonderful man was found to have incurable colon cancer. During his first hospitalization for treatment of the cancer, he read the *New York Sunday Times* review of Bernie Siegel M.D.'s first book, *Love, Medicine and Miracles,* (Harper Perennial, 60th Ed, 1998). After we began to work together again, he told me about Bernie's groundbreaking work and of the time that they had spent together on the telephone. In his way of "never telling my patients what to do," he said, "I strongly recommend that you get the book, read it, and meet the author." Within one week, I had bought a copy, read it, and found a workshop with Bernie in Watertown, Massachusetts.

At the workshop one month later, I heard Bernie describe his experience with what he called "support groups", a new term for me. I talked with the staff people about these support groups, and they suggested I become familiar with the work of Jerry Jampolsky, M.D. who would be giving a workshop there in Watertown the following month. I signed up for the workshop, where I heard Jerry describe his "Attitudinal Healing" groups. For these two fine physicians, the groups were open, loving forums in which people supported each other in their lives. I was long familiar with this kind of support on a one-to-one basis, and the idea of doing it in groups was wonderful. I could see that I could incorporate this kind of group in my practice. In less than two months, the first group consisting of five of my patients with cancer came together like magic.

Siegel felt that the most important healing attitude in his groups was *hope*. He would have liked to have called his groups "H.O.P.E. groups", and he felt that it would be important that the word, *hope*, be an acronym, H.O.P.E. However, with the exception of "E" for *Exceptional*, he could not decide on the words that would fit the acronym, so he chose to stay with the name that he had originally chosen, ECaP, which stood for, "Exceptional Cancer Patients".

In the first meeting of the group that came together out of my practice, I told them of my experiences with Siegel and Jampolsky. When they chose to keep meeting, I asked them if they would like to call themselves a H.O.P.E. group, telling them of Bernie's struggle with the hope acronym. When they enthusiastically agreed, I suggested that in all fairness to Bernie, the name was theirs only on the condition they figure out what the letters stood for. When we came together the next week, I asked them if anyone had come up with the words for the acronym. Sharon Williams, RN, an operating room nurse with whom I had worked for years, and who also conducted the *I Can Cope*[xv] group in our hospital, shyly raised her hand and offered, "*Healing Of Persons Exceptional?*" Sharon had given me a lot of help and encouragement in developing the group and, and now she was naming it. They loved it.[xvi]

That first H.O.P.E. Group met on February 12, 1987. It was a memorable occasion. The rest of 1987 would prove to be a memorable year for me in many other ways. One month later, I heard for the first time a song by the Grateful Dead called *Ripple*. I was fascinated by the lyrics to this simple tune with a funky country and western beat. It took me a few more weeks to find a copy of it, and I felt that the song would be a good convocation for our H.O.P.E. group meetings. The H.O.P.E'rs loved the words to that song and we sang it at the beginning of every meeting until the Grateful Dead began to become a thing of the past, and we had devised and published a convocation that clearly set the context of every H.O.P.E. Group meeting.

With the frequent repetition of the word, "ripple", I began flashing back to my last memory in the "near drowning" that happened when I was about four years old. (p.p. 30–31). I later gave my mother plenty of opportunities in which to remind me that I had nearly drowned then and certainly would have if her sister "hadn't run into the water in her best summer dress, and rescued me". It took years before I would walk into water over my knees, and even more years before I would put my head underwater for any time at all. However, I could never get past my last memory of the episode, which was *peacefully*, *fearlessly* looking up at the shiny silver ripples in the surface of the water over my head

I became increasingly frustrated over the fact that I could not remember anything that happened after seeing those ripples. At that time there was a growing public interest in doing "inner child work". And coincidentally (?) as I was flashing back to those ripples, I received a promotional brochure for a workshop called *The Use of Metaphors in Healing the Wounded Child Within* given by a New Zealand-born psychologist, David Groves. I was drawn to it like iron filings to a magnet. There, David told us about memories that hide behind "metaphors" that take us up to, but not into, a traumatic event. I knew with perfect clarity what he was talking about. And when he asked if any of us had such a memory, my hand shot up, and he asked me to tell the group about it. When I came to the part about seeing those shiny ripples over my head, I paused, and he asked, "And what do the ripples know about what happens next?"

Suddenly, I was surrounded by crashing, splashing sounds, and I felt the pressure of two huge hands around my chest. "The ripples know *'Boom!'*" I choked.

"And what does *'Boom'* know about the ripples?" he asked.

"They're down there." I answered, looking down to my right at the splashing ripples that I could now see so clearly... right there in the conference room. I could also see the rake, metal end submerged, floating away from me.

"And what happens next?" came from David.

I felt myself spinning around in midair, seized again around my chest by those huge hands, and given a good shake. "It's my aunt!" I muttered in terror as I saw her mouth open and heard her holler, "Toby, you stupid little boy!"

As I write these words, their punishing condemnation still penetrates to the core of my being, more than two decades after I gave myself permission to finally hear them. I still *feel* the terror I knew back then both in 1937 and 1987.

I know now why I have such a powerful aversion to loud, insulting, deprecating words, especially "stupid". I *hate* it when people put down others for their stupidity, and I know why I paradoxically tend to put down people for doing "stupid" things. I know now why I had a frustrating and uncontrollable habit of setting myself up for making people angry with me and calling me "stupid." I was trying to heal that wound way down in my subconscious. I was hoping that person to whom I had just done something "stupid" would feel my anguish and forgive me. It took getting the memory back to bring about the forgiveness, the *letting go* of the terror that seized both of us.

In that magical instant in David Groves' workshop, I knew why my aunt was so angry... her older sister's only son had slipped away from her supervision and had nearly drowned. I understood it all at a profound and fundamental level. I never again set up situations in which I would get people angry with me for being stupid.

I also stopped being an angry man. I had used anger to intimidate people so they would not raise their voices at me. When they finally broke through my anger with theirs, I would become speechless and tremble in terror inside because I would be "stupid" once again. I would dissociate right in front of them, causing them to turn away from me in confusion and anger, when all I wanted was to hear my aunt Brunie say, "There, little Toby, you're all right."

I am fully aware that I have just given you examples of repressed memory, dysfunctional behaviors, and post-dramatic stress disorder from my own experience of life. The phenomenon of repressed memory is hotly debated today because there are no guarantees that the recovered memory is valid, resulting in false accusation of alleged perpetrators. From my own experience, several things attribute to the validity of this memory: First, my mother told me hundreds of times about something that had happened to me to which she was a witness. Second, when I recovered the memory, all blame and guilt evaporated in a deeply felt sense of relief and forgiveness that included both my aunt and me. Third, two dysfunctional behaviors, dissociation on the one hand, and creating serious angry encounters on the other, simply evaporated. Fourth, I acquired beneficial functional insights into myself, *as a person*. In short, the only effects of the recovery of the memory of this trauma were beneficial.

Perhaps the work of recovering repressed memories can proceed with greater safety if such benefit-seeking aspects can be derived from it. I teach those who guide H.O.P.E. Groups that there is but one criterion of success to apply to recovering repressed memories: the discovery of inner peace arising from compassionate forgiveness of both victim and perpetrator. There is no doubt in my mind that, given the opportunity to relive the most terrifying event of my life, *and keep it all in my conscious mind*, relieved me of my own post-traumatic stress disorder and its associated dysfunctional behaviors. I also believe that the fact that I could tell it to a group of people with whom I felt safe was an essential component to the entire healing process. In my case, the safe place was David Groves' workshop. In the case of those with whom I work, the safe place is either in my office, a H.O.P.E. Group, or a small group in a Circling the Soul workshop.

This experience had a profound ameliorating effect on the anger that had come close to killing me in 1972. I became aware that that accident was the result of the destructive power of my anger. I had felt a lot of guilt about the accident because I knew I had brought it on myself. Now I was able to let that guilt go and become fully responsible for having created the situation. That included the destructive words that I repeated twice daily for months before the accident.

I had learned from Nightingale and his friends that my words, "You're killing yourself, Ken," were an *affirmation* that empowered an *intention*. For years, I felt guilty for having created a self-fulfilling prophecy. It was not a good feeling to look back at the many ways my thoughts and emotions had created the accident. After Groves' workshop, that guilt evaporated in that rich experience of compassionate forgiveness.

I knew that I had literally "created my own reality" with my thoughts and their corresponding emotions as expressed in my intentional affirmations. I subsequently vowed I would pay much closer attention to the exact meaning of each word I used. People began to call me a "wordsmith" because I would call their attention to the implications of the words and phrases they used to describe themselves and others. I would do what I could to keep them from hurting themselves or others.

My metamorphosis

As the years went by, and the H.O.P.E. Group work developed, I found out a lot more about the power of the mind to create and hold an intention that is in effect a super goal. Being less judgmental and critical, I could look back at my life and find three significant experiences in which I exercised that power:

First, when I was about eleven years old, I set that intention to learn what love was that I described on page 42. I have been told repeatedly that H.O.P.E. groups are safe places of unconditional love, and these wonderfully affirming responses, repeated many times, show me that I have connected to my youthful intention.

Second, I intended to become a physician. I knew I had to work through the trauma of my mother's hurtful question about my ability to love and my introverted, sensing nature. I lost my sense of self-worth. I slid into a state that took me from being top of my class in grade school to the bottom of my class in college. It was a process that took ten years to complete. Halfway through it, though, I somehow knew with crystal clarity that the only profession for me was medicine, thanks to Kendall Kent Kane (p.36). It certainly had a lot to do with the fact that my father, his mother, and his older sister were Christian Scientists. And my mother came from a family of physicians. I know that sounds crazy, but that is how my family was. So how much of this intention was a product of my genes, my nature, my environment, my nurture, cannot be clearly established. When I couple all that with a passion to fix things, a pair of good hands, and a high mechanical attitude, I had to become a surgeon!

Third, I joined my wife in a complex intention of where we wanted to live after residency and military service. We had met during my student years and we got married at the end of my internship. Together, we went to Iowa City, Iowa, for my residency in general surgery. We decided we wanted to live in "a rural or semi-rural location with hills, trees, and four seasons" that had to be "within an hour of the ocean." And where we live today in semi-rural, hilly, four-seasoned Maine is a fifty-five-minute drive to the nearest access to saltwater.

As I was moving into a disastrous senior year in college, I *knew* that I was to become a physician and I committed myself to doing whatever was needed to get into medical school. The only school I had in mind was the College of Medicine at McGill University in Montreal, Canada. I wrote the Dean, got an appointment with him, and my father gave me a round-trip ticket to Montreal. (The details of that story lie on pp. 38-40.)

Flying back home, I had that stunning experience of seeing that gold-rimmed round opening in the thin higher layer of clouds (p. 40) I knew then that I did not have to go into the Army for two years. As soon as I got home, I told my father of the agreement between me and the Dean at McGill. My father responded beautifully by promising to pay my tuition to Rutgers University, Newark, provided they would take me as a day student – a fifteen-minute train commute. I applied, was accepted, got straight A's, and the Dean at McGill had an opening for me that fall. I did well at McGill, getting honors in several courses.

Many things have happened to me in my life, and even going back into childhood I have felt that many events, both painful and joyful, were so beautifully shaped and exquisitely timed that "co-incidence" seemed to be a way of dismissing the meaning in them. I learned early on not to go looking for the meaning because, eventually, it would come to me, often correcting my earlier search (and sometimes affirming it). I was even given help: my mother told me so often about that "near-drowning" that I can recall the details of it as if it were last week. I can remember seeing that garden rake leaning against the weathered, gray, clapboard wall of the cabin. I clearly recall hearing two voices inside speaking to me: one saying, "Oh, look at that nice rake! You can dig clams with that." and the other saying," Oh no, you can't, it's too wide and its teeth are too short." In the ensuing argument, one of the voices convinced me that I should take the rake and dig clams with it. By choosing to pick up that rake, I was given the challenge of my life. Without it, I would never have had this experience of life, nor would I have written this book.

To me, one of those two voices was my soul, and the other was my ego. Life is, as I have said, the journey of a soul. We can be conscious or unconscious of it. When we become conscious of it, we have recovered our soul, which is what this book is all about.

Chapter 6:
H.O.P.E.'s Legacy

Introducing the chapter...

"Legacy" means that, somehow or other, events from the past have come forward to the present influencing the way in which the future unfolds. It often happens that at the time the past comes forward, it is not immediately recognized for its source, but waits for a retrospective view. So, it is with my life, the elements of which comprise a story – my story. So, it is with H.O.P.E's story that grows out of mine.

H.O.P.E. came into being as a "supportive" group service for cancer patients in my general surgery practice on February 12, 1987. It grew out of an interaction of many legacies in my life. Its very existence comprised a flowing evolution during the quarter–century of its life to the present day that becomes a rich legacy of healing. The current seven – person leadership of H.O.P.E. have come to see it as a living entity helping all those humans it touches find meaning, value, and purpose in their lives.

At our first meeting, I told the group that Bernie Siegel had wanted to call his Exceptional Cancer Patients support groups "HOPE groups", but he said that he could not figure what the letters stood for. I asked the group if they would like to call themselves a H.O.P.E. Group, and they said "Yes". I said then that they would have to come up with what the letters stand for. At the next meeting, I asked them if they had come up with the acronym, and only one hand went up... the hand of the hospital nurse, Sharon Williams, who had earlier suggested that I could run a support group at Stephens Memorial Hospital. I asked her if she would share what she had, and she said, quite simply, "Healing of Persons Exceptional."

The group explored what the phrase meant, and we all agreed that "Healing" meant "becoming whole"; "Persons" was all of us; and "Exceptional" meant that no two of us were like... every one of us was an exception to everyone else.

The Story:

As I have said, I was born into a family of healers in 1933... medical doctors on my mother's side, and spiritual healers on my father's side. His mother and one of his two sisters were Christian Scientists and the other sister was Amy Gordon Hamilton, whose failure to respond to the Christian Science prayers to their "God" to stop her hemorrhaging led her to become a self-professed atheistic/agnostic Assistant Dean of the New York School of Social Work – a well-known social healer who loved human beings (personal communication).

In November 1954, it became clear to me that I was meant to have a career in medicine. I made an appointment with the Dean of the Faculty of Medicine of McGill University in Montréal, Canada, and negotiated the ways in which I would need to prove to the Dean that I was intelligent and capable of hard work. Flying home that day, the aircraft passed through one cloud layer to reveal another layer above it with a perfectly round hole to the West rimmed with golden light from the setting sun. I saw it as a sign that I was on the right path for my life. It gave me pause to realize then that I was living a directed life... the directions would come, and I only needed to pay attention to them and follow them.

I chose surgery in 1958 in the middle of my second year at McGill because I had a high mechanical aptitude and gentle, skilled hands. The Secretary to the Dean sensed my budding interest in surgery and offered me the opportunity to do a summer externship in surgery in Albuquerque, New Mexico, where McGill had a special relationship with the Bataan Memorial Methodist Hospital, providing four of its students the opportunity to get a first – hand experience with the practice of surgery. Normally McGill offered those externeships to third-year students but she felt the University would support making an exception for me because she felt it was appropriate for me to do this at this time., She did not know that I had accepted a summer 1959 position as a medical externe at the University Hospitals in Copenhagen, Denmark (another example of living my "directed life"). I accepted her offer, went to Albuquerque, and was assigned to a general surgeon, Joseph Garland Riley, M.D., who was a self-contained, skilled, gentle surgeon who showed me that a surgeon could enter the human body as if it were a temple... resolving a concern I had that surgeons might be like so many of the Montréal surgeons who had had coarse training in the WWII battlefields of Europe.

This "Directed Life" of mine had another experience that same summer that touched me deeply. I met a Diné woman at the Gallup Intertribal Ceremony. We connected instantaneously in a very comfortable, mutually supportive way that lives yet today. Friends at the Lovelace Clinic in Albuquerque invited me to go to Gallup for the experience of coming close to the First Nation People, specifically the Diné. On arrival, I went into the large exhibition hall filled with booths displaying the wares and skills of the People. The first one promoted appealing buckskin products. Interested, I went in and was greeted by a Diné woman dressed in native style. We struck up a conversation in which I told her why I was in Albuquerque, to which she replied, telling me that she was starting at Cornell Medical School in a couple of weeks. Well, the dialogue led me to offer her a ride to New York via my town, Short Hills, NJ. She accepted my offer, telling me that she as going up country with her fiancé and her mother, who could bring her to Albuquerque to where I was living.

There, we loaded up my little Chevy roadster and a three-day trip followed, in which we shared a lot of experiences, becoming fast friends. We stayed in touch through our respective medical educations: hers taking her as a primary care physician into a clinic in the Navaho Nation, and mine taking me into a small General Hospital in Norway, Maine. I became active in the practice of Holistic Medicine, and I accepted an invitation to take part in a holistic medicine conference in Scottsdale, AZ. I thought it would be great to visit my Diné friend by renting a car and driving through the Navaho nation to Albuquerque. I called her, and she asked if she could participate in the conference. I encouraged her to do so.

When I got to the Scottsdale conference center and registered, I went into the open area in the center of the motel. There, I sat down and engaged in chat with friends with the door to the lobby area directly behind me. Suddenly, I found myself saying softly, "She's here." I turned to face the door to the lobby just as she walked through it, heading toward me!... a rich mystery that worked with exquisite precision. Because I had had other mysteries in my life, I accepted this one with a deep inner sense of pleasure, never bored, always delighted, standing in awe at Life and how It works. I was deeply grateful that

Life had treated me so generously. We enjoyed each other's company for the duration of the conference, saying our "goodbyes" next to our vehicles in the parking lot.

We stay in touch. Her 2020 Holiday Greetings update letter arrived Christmas eve with these closing words, "I keep thinking Mother Earth is getting tired of being abused and wants to rid herself of us." My sympathies precisely stimulating me to do my very best to help humanity get on with its life.

I went to Copenhagen in the summer after the Scottsdale conference, as planned. There, through a remarkable event effected by a letter from my mother, I met and fell in love with the woman who would join me in marriage two years later, and with whom I live to this day. She would come to Montréal in time for my 1960 graduation from McGill, and we would marry a year later at the end of a rotating internship – my first year of residency training.

I found a powerful desire to do a second year of residency – this time in internal medicine – before starting my surgical residency. I stayed in the hospital of my internship, and, during a three-month neurology rotation, I worked under a Fellow in Neurology who was an American completing requirements for his neurosurgical board certification. That man, Joseph Keith, Jr, M.D., knowing that I had a sincere interest in becoming a rural general surgeon surgical suggested the residency at the University Hospitals in Iowa City, Iowa. I sent away for information about that program; liked it; applied for it; and was accepted. Following "Directions" again.

I started that residency in 1962, aware that the University of Iowa specialized in training rural surgeons, without questioning the implications of "rural". However, suffering from the heat of a steamy-hot, Iowa-August day in 1965, my wife and I set a joint intention to live and practice in a rural or semirural locale where there were four seasons (unlike Iowa's two), hills, and trees... all within an hour of the ocean. That intention was realized in 1970 after serving the US Army in Germany as a general surgeon. While they were overseas, my Christian Science healer aunt died and left us a home to return to in the Eastern Adirondacks... four hours from the ocean.

I went to work there in the Emergency Room of the local 23-bed hospital, and, on my first day there, I read a classified ad for a general surgeon to work in a semi-rural Maine hospital that was 40 miles from the ocean. I saw that it perfectly fit that 1965 intention; so, I sent in my resume. We were invited to an interview at Stephens Memorial Hospital in Norway, Maine. We felt attracted to the hospital and the region, and my application was accepted... my Iowa residency was just what was needed there in rural Maine.

I started my surgical practice in January 1971. Shortly thereafter, I became known as the doctor who listens because one of my early patients asked me if she could tell me a story about her life that she had never told anyone else, because she was going to have a major operation – her first – the following day and she thought it important to share her story. It was a story of sexual abuse as a girl and a young woman... no diagnosis possible... only open, uncritical listening. Somehow, I knew how to listen, because she said, when finished, "Thanks for listenin', Doc. Now I think I'm ready for tomorrow's operation." She was. She sailed through it.

In 1972, however, exhausted from saying "Yes" too many times, I crashed, *literally and figuratively,* as I described in the last chapter. Thirteen days in the hospital with a broken back and right ankle gave me time to consider that I had brought on the accident myself. It was a wakeup call to deal with a family anger issue that would take the next fifteen years to resolve through a variety of life situations, the first of which arose in 1975.

Then, confronted by a world that seemed angry at me, I complained about it to my practice manager, who promptly introduced me to the work of Earl Nightingale (http://www.nightingale.com/authors/earl-nightingale.html) that focused on sharing a life of learning the "essence of success," Nightingale's definition of which was "the progressive realization of a worthy ideal". Nightingale's lifetime studies showed me that we are all born with that worthy ideal, but life may have caused us to stray from it – even forget it – lost behind attitudes developed in response to an early – and manipulative – environment. Nightingale's lifetime of study had showed me that remembering and serving that "worthy ideal" was the single most healthy move a person could make in their entire lifetime, and that their *attitude* was the key to recovering it.

What Nightingale called the "Law of Correspondence" indicated that the anger I was seeing reflected my own anger. Nightingale had pointed out that that anger was the result of an earlier choice in one's lifetime, and, because it was not working now, it was time to choose anew. For me, the new choice was, "Take it easy, Ken." With that change of attitude, the anger faded from my environment. As circumstance would have it, the very next patient who told a story of suffering anchored it in an environment of anger – hers and her abuser's – and I could share what I had learned from Nightingale for her benefit. I subscribed to the monthly Nightingale–Conant *INSIGHT* audiotape series that would continue to provide me with helpful insights and guiding principles for my patients – and for me – for the next twenty years. This immensely rich experience became the foundation of H.O.P.E's work in and with "Attitudinal Healing," none of which could be found in my medical school curriculum or other postgraduate studies.

In 1985, intrigued by the power of this attitudinal work, I confided in a social worker friend that I was thinking of taking a two-year sabbatical to get a degree in psychology. She discouraged me from that because she sensed that the obligatory study of statistics would be a waste of time for me. In response to my request for an alternative, she introduced me to Rev. Barry Wood, M.D. – psychiatrist extraordinaire – who practiced in nearby Portland. She had a strong sense that the "chemistry" between us would be healthy, constructive, and creative. It was, and over the next eighteen months, Wood helped me become acquainted with my demons – showing me that the Greek word, "daemon" actually meant "guide". This introduced a core element of H.O.P.E's work – *confront your demon and it will have to guide you through its challenges*. Wood also taught me the dynamics of the attitudes of anger, fear, and love in terms of Karen Horney's psychology of moves: towards (loving), against (angry), and away from (fearful).

Through Wood, I met group work in the form of the twelve – step program. I had codependent issues in the relationship with my mother and her patterns of woundedness and shame for her wounds. This helped deepen my awareness of psycho–spiritual wounds and the attitudes that make such wounds, all of which assumed powerful roles in the development of H.O.P.E's work.

In 1986, Barry Wood was found to have an incurable colon cancer... just at the time when Bernie Siegel's book, *Love, Medicine, and Miracles,* was published and reviewed in the Sunday *New York Times* book review that Wood loved to read. Wood and Siegel got to know each other, and when I came back to work with Wood, Wood suggested that I "get the book, read it, and meet the author". I did and met Siegel at one of his "Psychology of Illness and Art of Healing" workshops one month later on a weekend that "just happened to be" when I was not on call. Siegel was teaching people about his work in "ECaP"(Exceptional Cancer Patients) support groups. I added this work to my twelve – step experiences, with Siegel introducing me to the practice of guided imagery, of which he was already a master.

During that weekend, Siegel's hosts told me about the work of the California psychiatrist, Gerald "Jerry" Jampolsky, M.D., who had convened the first "Attitudinal Healing" groups for children with life-threatening illnesses. As Life would have it, Jampolsky was to be hosted by the same people four weeks later – a weekend when I was again not scheduled to be on call. I signed up and met Jerry and his partner, Diane Cirincione, PhD, and their work.

The time was now December, 1986, and Sharon Williams, RN, the nurse at Stephens Memorial Hospital who had introduced me to Bernie Siegel,, asked me to teach the American Cancer Society program, "I Can Cope," to a group of Stephens Hospital patients recently diagnosed with cancer. I agreed, and, near the end of the course, Williams told me that members of the group wanted to continue to meet with me as a group. I was confident that I had the resources to be able to respond favorably to her request. At the same time, I found that five of my patients with cancer wanted to continue to explore life with me, reminding me of my experience in second year of medical school when I and my classmates were told that we were not going to be taught prognosis "because you do not have the right to limit your patient's life." Rather, we had the responsibility to "involve (our) patents in an understanding of their disease process, and, if serious, advise them to get their affairs in order and get on with their lives." The professor added one final instruction, "Then promise them that, as their physician, you will do everything in your power to help them get on with their lives."

At the first meeting of the group, I asked the members if they wanted to continue. Their affirmative reply led me to repeat Siegel's statement that he wanted to call his ECaP (Exceptional Cancer Patients) groups H.O.P.E. groups, but he could not figure out what the letters stood for. I asked my group if they wanted to call themselves a H.O.P.E. group, and, in response to their affirmation, I told them that they would have to figure out what the letters stood for. The very next week, Sharon Williams came to the meeting with the suggestion, "Healing of Persons Exceptional," which was met with energetic approval by everyone in the group.

The jewel now had a perfect setting: "Healing" was about gathering all of one's scattered life – fragments into one whole being. "Persons" spoke to their common, shared human – ness; and "Exceptional" spoke to the fact that no two human beings are alike... each is an exception to the other. Now it needed the marketing skills of an expert... and she came along seven months later: Christiane Northrup, M.D. She had heard of my H.O.P.E. group and wanted me to run one for her cancer patients. We had a charming and delightful 90–minute meeting in her office, after which I got on the road just after the passage of a strong late summer shower and found myself staring at a double–arch rainbow whose ends lay on two lovely, green hills... a sign similar to the golden circle I had seen in the cloud flying home from Montréal 33 years earlier. This would become H.O.P.E's logo.

Northrup arranged for space and time at Portland's Mercy Hospital, and fifteen of her patients came to the first meeting.... promotion had begun. Six months later, in response to a request for me to conduct yet another H.O.P.E. group – the fifth – I knew I had to choose between surgery and H.O.P.E. I had met two perfectly qualified general surgeons to continue the general surgical service at Stephens Memorial Hospital. I was free to follow H.O.P.E's call. Registering H.O.P.E. as a 501(c)(3) not-for-profit organization followed immediately.

Shortly after Northrup's call, I received an invitation to participate in an Elizabeth Kübler–Ross intensive workshop in southern Maine where I heard her tell the story of the legacy of butterflies – a European mythological symbol of miracle – that children marked for death in a Nazi concentration camp used their fingernails to scratch into every surface of the wooden barracks they were taken to the night that they were to die…. Now the elements of the H.O.P.E. logo had gathered themselves for one of the members of my first H.O.P.E. group – Ruth Dullea – to put together in a single piece of art that is H.O.P.E's registered logo today.

Northrup introduced me to the American Holistic Medical Association, in which I was active for a dozen years exploring the relationship between the H.O.P.E. work and my chosen profession. I maintained a sense that "holistic" implied the existence of a healthy attitude serving as the context for all forms of healthcare. Several of the founding members of that organization told me that they had supported this perception from its inception. That perception still holds true in the face of an almost overwhelming focus on the *technology* of disease treatment in the hands of a profession that, today, belies the rubric – "Healthcare".

In 1988, I made the acquaintance of a family practitioner of holistic medicine, John Randall, M.D., who served as a hypnotherapist working with women in obstructed labor because the opening of the uterus would not relax, even after hours of strong contractions. Through the process of hypnotic regression, he found that all of these women had been sexually abused in their early teen years. Through further gentle hypnotic suggestion, these women were able to relax the uterine cervix, permitting normal delivery. In this way, Randall helped me understand the nature of my mother's shame that underlay a complex pattern of addictive behaviors that were the reason for delivering me by cesarean section in 1933. It also helped me appreciate the spiritual nature of the requests for me to listen to women's stories of abuse.

In 1992 Lonise Bias came to Norway, Maine, to speak to the students of the middle and high schools about her perception, "All harm comes from the misapplication of knowledge." I spent private time with her listening to the story behind her belief that came from the tragic deaths of two of her sons: one as a result of cocaine used in the *misapplication* of his own knowledge and the other son murdered as a result of another person *misapplying* his knowledge. The story of that murder included hearing the voice of the second dead son at his wake telling her – from the other side – "Ma, I'm all right Ma. Nothing's ever wasted"…a story that has found meaning in all H.O.P.E. groups.

In 1993, in a quiet and peaceful Sunday morning meditation, I became aware of ten phrases that I knew described the function of a H.O.P.E. Group meeting. They comprised responses to four "success questions" I had developed out of my experience with Earl Nightingale's work: "Who are we?" "Why are we here?" "How are we going to get what we came for?" "What are we going to do with it when we have it?" I sensed that they were to be read at the beginning of every H.O.P.E. group meeting. They came to comprise the first page of a H.O.P.E. booklet called "The GoldBook" (because it was printed at the outset on goldenrod – – colored paper). My studies of Nightingale led me to know that those four questions were very neutral... useful to the good and the bad alike. His acquaintance with Jampolsky's work led me to know that Jerry's twelve "Principles of Attitudinal Healing" set a healthy, loving, compassionate, and forgiving context for what could be well recognized as a "business plan" for any life. Those principles became the second page of the booklet. I derived ten "Guidelines" for the conduct of a H.O.P.E. Group meeting from studies of other groups, particularly Jampolsky's, which, with the "Prayer for Serenity", comprised the third page. The fourth page to come to my mind was the title page, "H.O.P.E. Group Opening."

It became clear to me that this comprised an *alchemical* process which could be called a "H.O.P.E. Group". The function of any "H.O.P.E. Group" was to bring together all of the experiences of the participants in a fashion that created an alloy of thought from which every participant could take a portion for their own use, the experience of which they would bring back to the next week's H.O.P.E. Group meeting. I saw that the three components created a *crucible* for the meeting, and reciting the Prayer for Serenity at the end of the meeting would break the crucible in order for a new crucible to come into being at the next meeting... the alchemy of H.O.P.E.

In 1993, I met Margot Fanger, MA, LCSW, at a conference on consciousness, and we became fast friends, with Fanger contributing significantly to H.O.P.E's experience with the conduct of H.O.P.E. Group meetings. She saw that the role of the person that could be said to be in charge of the meeting was not that of a "facilitator" because the work in a H.O.P.E. Group was not to make things easy, but to help people challenge their demons to help reveal those personal resources that would get them through their most difficult challenges. To Fanger, the role of "leadership" was synonymous with Robert Greenleaf's concept of "Servant Leadership," implying that H.O.P.E. Group "leadership" was more that of a "guide" than a "facilitator", or coach.

In 2005, moved by the spiritual nature of a H.O.P.E. Group meeting ascribed to by its participants and the story of the children and the images of butterflies, I looked into the remarkable phenomenon of metamorphosis. As part of my study, I found out that the Ancient and Modern Greek word for butterfly is Psyche... the same as their word for soul! Investigating further, I found that the belief in the soul was destroyed in the early part of the seventeenth century by the French Rationalists who believed that unless the existence of any phenomenon or concept could be scientifically proven, it did not exist! Further study revealed that the death of the soul at that time was simply the beginning of a hibernation that ended at the end of the twentieth century with the appearance of a plethora of books relating to the soul. My studies showed me that soul is not synonymous with mind or spirit. Rather, it is the bridge between the two and it is that which dissociates near death and subsequently reincarnates. This larger and deeply mystical appreciation of our spiritual nature is another facet in the jewel – like foundation of H.O.P.E... with profound implications for our potential.

In 2008, I was traveling home with Onani Meg Carver, MA, a gifted healer from the Ojibwe traditions who had come together with me at a conference in consciousness in 2007 where we were invited to co – chair the 2009 conference. She told me how she had used her healing practice to make a deep cut in a finger *disappear* in 15 minutes. In answer to my, "How, Meg?" she said, "By being present and letting go of fear." This, in turn, encouraged me to investigate the power of *presence*. My studies led me to Joseph Campbell's quote of the twelfth century Hermeticist, Alain de Lille: "God is an intelligible sphere whose center is everywhere and whose circumference is nowhere." This reminded me of Albert Einstein's perception that every point in the universe is at the exact center of its universe. Einstein and others of his ilk made the point that it is impossible to get outside the universe to study it, and it could only be measured in terms of its relationships *within* itself. I was reminded that Sogyal Rinpoche in his 1992 Harper Collins book, *The Tibetan Book of Living and Dying,* maintained that fear is a projection from the present to a time that does not exist and anger is a projection from one's own center to a space that does not exist for the angry one, making both fear and anger *illusions.* The Rinpoche said further that removing those projections would transform fear into *awareness* and anger into *presence.* Meg's cut was the result of both fear and anger, and though it may seem like a stretch, it was an *illusion* from which she could free herself by letting go of that fear... using methods she had learned from her Ojibwe healer – teacher during a ten – year apprenticeship.

In the last four years, I have been reading sources giving the evidence for our universe evolving 13.7 billion years ago from that point of light called the "Big Bang". These sources shared the perception that our universe came into being as a manifestation of a dimensionless field of consciousness. That evolution has been extremely powerful but not violent in the way that we humans use violence to kill each other – from fear. Rather, its violence is, in and of itself, fearlessly creative... when the Universe turns a star into a nova, it creates heavy elements. Those elements are the heavy elements in our bodies. Yes, friends, we are, indeed, "Star Dust" promised us from the beginning of time in that Big Bang.

When I read Nick Herbert's *Quantum Reality* (Anchor Books, 1985) in 1988, it gave me the opportunity to know that consciousness was a fundamental property of the tiniest particles of the universe, all of which had come into existence in the first few microseconds of the "Big Bang". This led me to develop a set of expressions that comprise the essence of H.O.P.E's work:

We have been promised these lives since the beginning of time. That beginning has a perfect integrity. It is the instantaneous product of a dimensionless field of consciousness. Our consciousness (mind) derives from that consciousness. The Universe has a body that becomes our bodies. We are alive because It is alive. It is defined by its relationships, as we are defined by the relationships of the 30 trillion cells that comprise every adult human body... their relationships are harmonious... they are love – compassionate, creative love. No two of us are alike. There is no divine hierarchical order separating human beings. Each one of us is a once – told tale, a once – sung song, a once – written novel, a once – read a poem, a once – danced dance... please tell me your tale; sing me your song; read me your novel; recite for me your poem; and dance for me your dance. You honor me. Thank you.

We now know that we are not accidents of a blind struggle for survival. We have not stolen knowledge; rather, it was given us without condition. This empowers us to accrue experience which shows us that in our perceived shame for having stolen knowledge from its Source, we have trudged out into an ever-deepening darkness *of our own choice*. Today, more than ever before, we are slowing down the trudge and raising our heads to see that the fading flickering light which illuminates our way comes from behind us. We are choosing to reverse course and go to the light that comes from our Source – a beacon calling us home – certain that Its direction gives us the power of peace that takes us to the stars in service of the Source, Itself.

In this way, the legacy that became H.O.P.E. over the last 40 years becomes, in turn, a legacy that helps us move forward through a deep forest of darkness to the light that shows us the way Home. H.O.P.E. chooses to participate in *our* metamorphosis.

Chapter 7:
What's Next (introductory thoughts)

Standing at a fork in our road facing our demons

In case you had not figured this out already, we are in chaos today. I liken it to standing at a fork in our road facing our demons. Like it or not the situation demands that we face our most powerful Demon, the Lord of Chaos, Satan, himself. The famed major league baseball player, Yogi Berra, tells us, "When you come to a fork in the road, take it." That being the case, where do the two branches of our fork take us? In our present state of affairs, I see the one branch leading down a barren road to a dusty death that could be nuclear. I see the other branch leading to a greening of the Earth Mother. If you have trouble understanding this, please be patient. Let me share what crosses my mind now, two important images: our limitless spiritual nature and the limited life span of all revolutions, two of which are in their death throes as we speak: the 18th century. industrial and political.

As a segue, I share with you my fascination with the universe that goes way back in my life. I grew up a few miles from the great Bell Telephone radio telescope that picked up the background radiation from the Big Bang. I visited it when I was a teenager. I was later fascinated by the quantum reality aspects of this universe; delighted to find out that it was finite, beginning as a point of light nearly 14 billion years ago. I was also fascinated to learn about the quantum experiments that proved that consciousness is a fundamental aspect of matter... and that matter is a fundamental aspect of consciousness. On the one hand, it was apparent that matter can be measured in terms of space and time. On the other, it was apparent that consciousness cannot be measured in terms of space and time... It is both infinite and eternal... everywhere... now!

As I said (p.73) "We have been promised these lives since the beginning of time." I was delighted to read in Peter Kingsley's marvelous work, *Reality* (The Golden Sufi Center, 2004), "We are immortal," appearing for the first time on page 520 of that 600-page book. I saw that he was leading up to it by the time I had reached page 40, and wondering where he would say it. Being immortal says something about our timelessness that I want the reader to take under serious consideration: the "stuff" that comprises us is 13.7 billion years old. It is not only finite space time but infinite, immeasurable consciousness.

About 25 years ago, a friend told me how he had a heart attack and, knowing that he had died, he went into a beautiful place of color, light, and love, knowing that he was dead. He was aware that a very important piece of creative work had been interrupted by his death and immediately he heard a voice saying that he was to go back and finish it. On returning to this life, he finished his work; told me about it; had a second heart attack; and left for good. He was the first of six people I have gotten to know who have had similar experiences with their own dying and going beyond their death. They all returned to complete an important service to others.

All of this makes perfect sense to me... not in terms of logical thinking, but knowing, as Antoine de St. Exupéry writes in his book, *The Little Prince,* "It is only with the heart that one can see rightly. The essential is invisible to the eye."

I recently finished reading Chris Hedges' *Wages of Rebellion* (Nation Books, 2015) in which he examines the nature of unsuccessful and successful revolutions. He finds that successful revolutions create their own "vocabulary" that the oligarchs, against whom they rebel, cannot understand. The unsuccessful revolutions fail to create such a vocabulary. As I went through this, I realized that every revolution has a lifespan, the end of which comprises a disintegration of the thought forms that had created the revolution. That disintegration is inevitably chaotic.

The chaos that we see around us today marks the ending of prior revolutions. Consider that the three revolutions of the 18th century are in their death throes as we speak. One of the revolutions is industrial and social: The Industrial Revolution of 1750. The other revolutions are political and social: the American Revolution of 1776 and the French Revolution of 1789. Fundamental to the vocabulary of the approaching revolution are words that reflect attitudes and belief systems. Examples of the former are kindness and compassion. Examples of the latter are all associated with globalization, which, to me, implies the growing recognition of our universal equality in the context of an immense diversity.

In respect to that image of universal equality as a reflection of the new vocabulary, there is a defensive, terribly fearful retreat into the dark side of the dying revolutions. In this way, I can begin to appreciate the behavior of a class of powerful individuals that now call themselves the Elite. This is not what you think it is; rather, it is the product of a denial that there are limited resources to keep us going in our consumption of those resources. There is a class of individuals who have accumulated great wealth from the consumption of our limited resources. They do not see that when we run out of these resources, all of us will suffer the same fate as any homeless human on the streets of every hometown. Yes, denial can take incredible forms… one only needs to be reminded of the Holocaust.

It occurs to me that the trillions of dollars accumulated by these ravenous, insatiable appetites represent the energy that can keep the earth and its human population very much alive and well. It occurs to me as well that it does not pay to try to isolate these highly creative and intelligent, but misguided, human beings. They will only retreat into their bomb shelters and hire mercenaries to protect them from what is really going on. Better to look peacefully at them in their fear and acknowledge it by saying, "I see what you want me to do, and I will not do it because I will not let you control my life and the lives of so many other real human beings. So, come out of your bomb shelters. We are not going to hurt you. Rather, we are going to follow the example of Bishop Desmond Tutu confronting the police lining the walls of his Grace Cathedral to prevent a march against apartheid. He extended his open hand, saying, "You cannot mock my God; for He cannot be mocked. Come join the winning side. You have lost already."

Do we not need H.O.P.E. Groups to help each other get through this time? H.O.P.E. groups, yes – any way, big or small, supportive of each other using a loving, gentle, non-judgmental approach to achieve unity instead of separation.

"The Great Secret" Reveals Itself in Our Longing

It is my sense of it all that we are moving into a space of solving what Peter Kingsley calls "The Great Secret[xvii]"… "Source" isn't where we think It is, out there. It is in here – within you, me, everything – and continuously revealing

Itself to us… not so much through our rational, logical minds as through our senses and our intuition… our *longing*. Kingsley tells me that the ancient Greek prophets, Parmenides and Empedocles, were given the key to The Secret 2500 years ago. It was more than the later – Socratic – Greeks, could grasp. They've misled us into believing that we can know Source through rational and logical thought. The "Secret" is neither rational nor logical: it is a "Mystery" found only by going within to the depths of our sensing/feeling and intuition. So, maybe, just maybe, those feelings you may feel: fear, anger, shame, blame, and guilt, for instance, are invitations to go to those depths and find that you are not alone, as the man in the first story below discovered in his Hanoi Hilton imprisonment. You are never alone in your deep longing and when you own that, the door to the Mystery opens. Here are five stories of people who found and followed their deep longing; and none of them were ever alone after the Mystery revealed itself to them[xviii].

A Navy F4 Phantom pilot flying a combat mission early in the Vietnam conflict got shot down over Hanoi. His ejection – seat parachute saved his life, but he was captured and sentenced to isolation in the prison that came to be known as the "Hanoi Hilton". His isolation was so extreme that he felt he would either go mad or die. Facing those fears, he developed a determination to meditate deeply and regularly to "find myself" (as I later heard him say). When he finally found himself, he became aware that he "was not alone." As I listened to his account, I got the sense that he became aware of the longing that we all have and have always had: to know that Mystery and live it because it has always been with us.

Peter Kingsley, early in his college years, went to a bookstore looking for an interesting book. A book jumped off a shelf onto the floor at his feet, open; so, he picked it up and read what it had opened to. It became a clear – cut instruction for him to study the works of the prophets, Empedocles and Parmenides. (If you should be curious, go visit http://peterkingsley.org . You will see where his longing has taken him.)

I, Ken, your author, having grown up in a family of spiritual healers, allopathic healers, and atheist social healers… am aware of my longing to help humans everywhere "get on with their lives". The longing has come to me several times in my life, weaving its way through a variety of situations. This time, I recalled it when I read the September 2006 Parabola essay, "As Far as Longing Can Reach"[xix] by Peter and Maria Kingsley. Several years ago, I had gone into a bookstore on 23 December to buy a Christmas present paperback for my wife that she said she wanted. The bookstore was crowded, and I did not know where to find the book; so, I started looking for a clerk. Due to the size of the crowd, progress was slow, and at one point, I found myself standing still next to a narrow display rack with shelves of paperbacks stretching from floor to ceiling. Suddenly, I saw a movement above me... a paperback jumping off the top shelf to land at my feet... the very book I was looking for!

Meg C, a close friend and colleague of Ojibwe extraction, who had been trained in the Ojibwe Midewiwin healing traditions, found herself in a stressful situation while she was slicing carrots in preparation for a meal. Momentarily distracted, she sliced a finger to the bone. She put pressure on the cut, stopping the bleeding. Her partner suggested they go to the hospital and get it sewn up. She responded with, "Not now, I have work to do." She became "present and let go of all fear". Fifteen minutes later, aware that the "work" was done, she took the pressure off and there was no sign that the finger had ever been cut! When she told me that story, she showed me the finger... there was no scar. With this, she knew she was being called to practice her native ways – her longing – and was able to successfully combine the practice and raise a family.

Evy M, a graduate nurse in a teaching hospital, developed a symmetrical weakness of her arms that became an aggressive form of ALS (Lou Gehrig's disease). When the paralysis put her in a wheelchair with useless arms and legs, she saw herself in the full-length mirror in her hospital room and said to her reflection, "God, Evy, how I hate you!" She had been deformed by polio in her youth, and always had a limp and could never find clothes that fit properly but had never acknowledged self-hatred. She swore then that she would not die hating herself, and, because "love" was the opposite of "hate," she was determined to come to love herself completely before she died. It was a difficult and challenging process that involved looking at her naked body in that mirror every day for one whole hour and extending love into it. It took several weeks. When it was nearly complete, she stopped, wondering if coming to *love* herself completely was going require her to *like* the disease that was killing her. She persisted, and when the love was complete, she no longer identified herself with her disease! The disease progressed over the next week or so to the point where she had the strength to breathe for no more than ten minutes... she stayed in that state for 36 hours! Then, to her surprise, having accepted her death with grace, her strength began to return! It took two full years for the recovery to complete itself. She knew then that it was time to change her career and go into the one that she had always wanted – a Christian ministry. It was successful, and she went on to become the ordained Methodist minister of a parish in Newburgh, New York. She had found her longing and had followed it. She lived for many more years in good health. I have not heard from her since 2008. Very recently, though, I found the courage to exercise my curiosity and contacted her old Parish. They told me that she had developed a benign health condition that made it necessary for her to move to the Southwest. She's alive and well today.

I found the Kingsleys' *Parabola* essay yesterday and sensed it was what I'd been looking for as context for this blog. Am I surprised? I am delighted.... It is my sense today that we are moving into a time of breaking open "The Great Secret"... Source has its own longing... to be intimately known by all sentient beings... including humans.... it has imbued itself in you, in me... in everything. The "Secret" isn't a secret... It is the great Mystery of the One.

I offer you these questions: Are not fear, depression, and anxiety all expressions of a deeper, oh-so-very human longing? Has that longing not been with us forever? Is it not to be found in the works of poets, artists, composers? Do we not flood ourselves with ever more distractions today, smiling whitely during an epidemic of violence in a myriad of ugliness that rises out of our own longings? Is this not what underlies addictions and suicide? Are we not like the solitary rat in a cage choosing cocaine-laden water over unmedicated water, who stops the cocaine choice within days after a second rat is put in the same cage with the same choice of waters? Are we not exploring what motivates the suffering of the world today and finding it to be a longing to be close to Source and Source's own great longing to be known and loved by us, the product of Its divine imagination?

Finally, could it be that Source was at work with its own longing when it expressed itself through the remarkable (and improbable) life of Stephen

Hawking? Could it be that Source was at work with Its own longing when It expressed Itself through the remarkable, one–of–a–kind life It gave you?

Quartets

I dedicate this concept to the three who came together in the first "Quartet": Elaine M, Berry M, and Jacob W, whose idea it was to think of the value of meetings in fours – "Quartets". We had come together to share our spiritual outlook(s) on life. We agreed that this meeting was loving, nurturing, kind, and creative.

Those of you who know me and the way I have experienced life... not as something that I went out and looked for, but something that came with assignments for me. This simple principle is common to spiritual practices. My life has been a directed life since as far back as I can remember. Twice within but a few months, I was one of four people to come together to explore our creative nature rich in these values: loving kindness, care, compassion, creativity, meaning, value, and purpose. These two occasions had no one in common except me.

The first meeting came about as two old friends – women I have known for years – and I started to talk about coming together for a noon meal in their city, Portland. As this dialogue began, I received a call from an old friend – a man I had not seen for a couple of years – asking me if we could get together for a noon meal at a good family restaurant about halfway between the two cities where we live. I mentioned the meeting I was going to have with these two women, and he wondered if it would be possible for him to join us. I told him I would ask my friends if he would be welcome. They were pleased to have him join us... they had their own experience of him and his ministerial career.

We had a richly creative and comfortable lunch together in Portland. At the end of our meal, he commented on the fact that we were a "Quartet", the dynamic of which he considered to be balanced and pleasantly creative. We committed to having another such time together in the future... no specific day set.

Shortly after that fine meeting, three people appeared in my life, none of whom knew me or each other. They were called together by the organization I started in my surgical practice in 1987, H.O.P.E, through its website, https://hopehealing.org . They announced their presence and their curiosity all within a few days of each other. What we had in common, moreover, was a powerful interest in helping human beings develop beyond our old limited and selfishly egocentric thinking. After experiencing a series of dialogues between us as individuals we decided to come together in a longer dialogue comprising all four of us using the communication vehicle, ZOOM, which made it possible for the four of us to meet: a creative businessman from New Jersey, an "evolved" businessman from Montréal, and a social worker in the school system of a suburb of Melbourne, Australia. We were curious about how it was that we all came together within a period of less than one week without any prior introductions. It became clear that through our differences we were to work with each other to improve the quality of our individual callings.

As we were planning this meeting, I was reminded of the Quartet that had met for lunch in Portland, and, to me, this was another "Quartet". Both of these Quartets had concerns for humanity, and I could see how the concept of "Quartet" could spread... and how rapidly! We talked about this rapid spread, and wondered what would happen if the four members of one Quartet each called together another Quartet to explore our human potential, thus bringing twelve new people into working together as Quartets. Each one of those could convene Quartets to explore a major shift in consciousness, becoming geometrically expanding to create a new civilization... one based on benefit – compassion, creativity, kindness, service, peace, love, etc.

Consider that the civilization which began with the Renaissance and reached its peak with the Industrial Revolution is now dying... as all civilizations die. Consider that the forces which created the past civilizations were ones that focused on ego – driven survival. Consider that what I am talking about is a natural component of evolution: spirit–driven thriving. Consider that the Mother Earth on which we live, and from which we derive our physical bodies, is not an accident, but the product of a field of consciousness that comprises and involves the entire universe, just as the field of space – time comprises and involves the entire universe.

Consider that the power figures of the old civilization are highly creative human beings who thrive on control by creating fear, shame, blame, and guilt throughout humanity. Consider that their leaders live in secret... a cabal who have profited greatly from war and consumption of natural resources. Consider the effect of an expanding field of consciousness comprised of countless millions of Quartets and the consciousness that convened them. Considered that this phenomenon has, like all other natural phenomena, a tipping point. Consider that the work of the Quartets is not any form of warfare and consumption... the creativity of the cabal would then be welcome in the creation of a completely new civilization.

Consider your potential to contribute to the new civilization... convene a Quartet.

A Trio of blogs

1-- Purification Time: an old Prophecy Coming True... but how? September 9, 2017

(It's all about remembering what we had forgotten: We Are Immortal)

I would like to start by introducing you to something about me that I suspect I share with a great many people, but that we seldom talk about. Before I had lived in this lifetime for five years, I knew that that which I grew up calling "God" loved me because it is love, and the story about God in the Garden of Eden could not be true. I knew that the loving God would never punish its children in the way stated in the legend. I had this thought as I was listening to my grandmother read me Genesis 3, which was part of the weekly Sunday morning scriptural lesson in her household. The thought stayed with me, guiding me through my life from its background over the next 80 – odd years.

This thought matured into a "knowing" when I was given a copy of Nick Herbert's 1985 book, *Quantum Reality* (Anchor, 2011) In it, I discovered that my universe had a beginning and that consciousness is a fundamental property of matter. This led me to an appreciation that I have been promised my life since the beginning of time, nearly 14 billion years ago!

I found that sharing that idea with people in my H.O.P.E. Groups helps them begin to see themselves differently – to be of greater value to self and others. To put it simply, I began to look at all of my knowing as, in fact, a "remembering". Indeed, what I am about to pursue with you are the implications of a tragic "forgetting" that has led us into a disastrous situation... a situation that, fortunately, is reversible. The process has its name – *Purification*.

Before we explore the concept of "Purification," I want to go a step further: We live in an expanding Universe which began as a point of light that comprised both matter and consciousness. As revolutionary as this may sound, the evidence for it is solid: we've found that the Universe is expanding from a beginning instant, and subatomic particles share information about each other as if time and space do not exist. (I invite you to visit these phenomena with the help of Google and all encyclopedias, like I did... yes, they are proven theories!)

Peter Kingsley, PhD. historian, a passionate devotee of the really ancient (pre-Socratic) Greeks, Empedocles, Parmenides, and Pythagoras, makes the simple statement of our immortality in his rich work, *"Reality"* (The Golden Sufi Center; First Edition, 2004). Kingsley opens *A Story Waiting to Pierce You*, (The Golden Sufi Center, 2010) with a two-sentence quote from the Hopi Elder, Thomas Banyacya, that come from a 1990 Beyond Words publication, *WISDOMKEEPERS:*

"If you don't stop what you're doing, Nature will intervene. Other forces far beyond your control will come into play. The last stages are here now.... Our Prophecies tell us in the last stages the White Man will steal our lands. It's all happening now. We pray and meditate and ask the Great Spirit to keep the world together a while longer. But it's coming. The Purifiers are coming."

I would add that there is a growing cadre of humans who are in communication with Great Spirit working to hold the world together. Please add your prayers to theirs. Thank you.

2. The Malignant Ego-Mind, April 12, 2020 (A real-life horror movie...)

I would like to share with you the thoughts that arose as I considered the implications of Easter in the Christian tradition. I got an Easter greeting from an old friend of mine and his lovely wife. He and I have shared some very rich experiences – some painful and some comforting –. Here are two of the opening thoughts they shared with me:

In this real-life horror movie in which we live today, we know there is a vicious creature we cannot see. But-because it is not causing any symptoms, it can secretly be living in anyone who is near us. Equally frightening, we know this virus can, suddenly, and-without any of us even being aware-fly into our lungs and kill us.

This is the horrible Good – Friday merry – go – round – ride on which we are all stuck. Nobody knows when it is going to stop, but Everybody knows that the triumphant positive energy of Easter comes next.

I offer you an image for your thoughts... the name for that vicious creature you (we) cannot see... "Wetiko", a thought form that is pure evil. The word comes from the Cree people and has a couple of analogues in other eastern tribes. Paul Levy translates that into "Malicious Egophrenia". If you're like me, "ego" is just what you think it is, and "phrenia" means "mind". The Eastern Natives saw that the coming white man was a devil in disguise with a nice song but murder in its mind. Wetiko stands for humans and their institutions that mindlessly destroy Mother Earth and her children. Look at our leadership....

I have been rereading a lot of Paul Levy's thoughts, and I realize that I learned much from him and my cousin Pat – a respected Jungian student-counsellor – quite a few years ago. I have carried this ego-mind concept in *my* mind in "guiding" 5,000-odd H.O.P.E. Group meetings where many people have surrendered to powerful egos, either their own or somebody else's. So, I take the twelve-step concept of ego and use their acronym, "Ease God Out" from the word that means "I". I was shown years ago that the ego needs the love and compassion of the spirit that shows us that my "I" is part of a spiritual collective known as "We". Dreams have shown me that my ego – my secular, DNA-related part of me – does not know why I was created, but my soul – my "higher" spiritual self – does know why it is here, having occupied other "human animal" bodies through their lifetimes.

73

I am of a clear mind that Jesus knew that he was taking on the Wetiko of society and he knew that he would have to give up his human body in order to start the healing metamorphosis. And the struggle goes on in the Amazon forests and in the minds of Monsanto and in a lot of what we call "politics" and even "medicine" today.

This is, indeed, a remarkable time in the life of humanity, and we might even sense a gratitude to COVID-19 for clearing our polluted air and our fearful minds.

Thank you for your thoughts, and the opportunity to re − examine those thoughts that I have just shared with you. If a dialogue grows out of this, so be it. I welcome it.

3. A Dream of the Future, March 13, 2015 (A "key" dream I had five years ago... about a train wreck that I saw happen, and the subsequent adventure that led to life showing me a beautifully clear image of where we humans are going.)

The Dream:

A good friend (my childhood alter ego, Rookie) had invited me to go with him on a drive down to the western shore of Penobscot Bay. This was an invitation that I could not refuse... it's a piece of God's country that I love to visit and then return home to another piece of God's country that nurtures me to the depth of my soul.

When we got to Pen Bay, he drove up to an outlook point and parked the car. We got out to take in the beautiful view. We had no sooner got to the berm overlooking the bay than I heard a loud racket off to my right. I turned to look at what could possibly be causing it, only to be frightened by the sight of a 1940's three car commuter train crashing through the dense woods, clearly off its track and seemingly without an engineer. It was going so fast that when it reached the berm it launched out over the bay, crashing into the water.

As it went past, I could see that it was full of passengers − very strange ones, indeed. They all looked alike: modern businessmen in black suits, with white shirt and dark tie; very fair skin and smoothly combed black hair. They looked like paper cutouts glued onto the glass of each window. Curious, I walked up to the train as the end was just about to disappear under water. Suddenly, a strange pale white porcelain – like hand reached out and grabbed me by my right ankle – the one that was distorted by a 1972 accident that had caused a lot of damage. Surprised, but fearlessly, I knew that my walking stick – an Irish shillelagh – would free me from that death grip. I reversed the shillelagh and smashed that porcelain hand.

As the train disappeared under the water, a huge, sightless, gray aquatic mammal rose out of the water and dropped itself down on the train, assuring the death of all its passengers. I felt a strong sense of relief as I saw this part of the dream come to its end. I looked across the wreckage of trees to see a dense, dark forest looming on the other side. I knew I had to go through it! I worked across the wreckage and stood looking at a standing tree, not knowing how to move from there. The tree began to glow, and I knew I had to ask it to help me find a way through. It told me to look past it and find the next glowing tree. I did, and in this way, tree by tree, I found my way through the forest.

When the forest began to brighten, I could see a clearing beyond it. When I entered the clearing, I found myself looking at a large railroad terminus with a three-car train on each track next to its platform. As I looked further, I saw people coming out of the forest, walking towards the platform directly in front of them. After climbing the short flight of stairs onto the platform they filed into the passenger cars. When a train was full of passengers, the doors closed and the train left the station. Looking farther ahead of the moving train, I could see that every track leading out of the terminal would join with all other tracks until there was but one track with all of the trains moving toward beautiful golden sun light on the horizon.

I knew I was looking at the future of the human race on earth.

Life gets my attention:

I thought I was done with the whole thing a year ago... nobody interested in taking the H.O.P.E. business to the larger audience. "Me?" I asked Life. "Yup," says she, breaking my right hip in its neck, dropping me to the floor in a world of hurt. Rather than going then to the hospital, I asked my wife to help me get upstairs into my bed. (Why, you ask? I live a directed life; so, read on.)

toughing it out overnight with the help of Aleve, I got to Stephens Hospital by ambulance the next morning, meeting a Swedish-trained orthopod who said, "You're lucky you have me. As opposed to your countrymen who make you recover for four months by not cementing the prosthesis in, I'm going to cement the prosthetic ball in place and you'll be up walking tomorrow." He was true to his word, and I was home in three days, during which time a dozen people I'd worked with came to visit – separately – and every one of them reminded me of the wonderful way I cared for my patients! Shucks, that was my passion that I'd found in second year of McGill Medicine: "Always promise your patients that you'll do everything in your power to help them get on with their lives."

What a reminder from Life that she was not done with me! Today we need to hear more humans saying to those who suffer that we can and will do everything in our power to help humanity get on with its life.

A shaman's journey:

As the title of this book implies, a metamorphosis in the life of the author that would that be expressed in the change from being a surgeon to that of being a shaman. I knew very little about shamans and shamanism when I went into surgery. When I started the H.O.P.E. Group in Portland in 1988, I was told by the participants that I had a quality that they had found in the work of Michael Harner, PhD. They strongly recommended that I read his book, *The Way of the Shaman* (HarperOne, 1990), because they felt that I would learn something about myself by reading it.

I did... and from reading his book, I saw that Shamanism is a worldwide practice, and, in many native societies, the shaman is the one who gets called before the medicine man. Shamanic work reveres the soul, finding it to be strong, personal, and yet fragile. In illness and trauma, the soul gets fragmented and the shaman is called to put the pieces back together. I had met "soul" many years before, but had never tried to learn anything of depth about it... too religious. Harner's work, "Core Shamanism" appealed to me, and in the next issue of the catalog from the Interface educational organization in a Boston suburb, I saw the announcement for a Core

Shamanism workshop by him. I signed up, and got a rich appreciation of this ancient practice, especially as brought forward into contemporary times.

I found I could easily enter a state of "non-ordinary, shamanic" consciousness that helped the person for whom I "journeyed" to seek answers to fearful questions... answers they could not find otherwise. I took training in shamanic journeying from Michael and I later took "soul retrieval" training from his student, Sandra Ingerman. I focused on shamanic work in my counseling practice in the late 1990s, and continue the practice to this day.

I cannot close this work without going on a personal shamanic journey with what is known as a "power animal" who is my "spirit guide" to help guide my practice. The animal that appeared to me in this journey had never served as my power animal before. I was surprised and delighted when a female mountain lion came into my imaging. This animal is enormously powerful... nurturing, peaceful, and courageous... qualities that I nurture in myself. She encouraged me to continue doing the work that I am doing and for writing the book about my journey. It is appropriate for helping others get on with their lives.

And with those encouraging thoughts, I continue my life with her courageous nature always at hand. I am aware this work might cause fear in some, and I can share her courageousness with them. I will close by saying that my service is the service of the female mountain lion, and I am open to all thoughts and questions.

Epilogue

Evolution

Isn't it about time we ended the violence?

Revelation: the Uncaused Cause has been revealing itself to us continuously. We have been promised these lives since the beginning of time. That beginning has a perfect integrity. It is the instantaneous product of a dimensionless field of consciousness. Our consciousness (mind) derives from that consciousness. The Universe has a finite, space-time body that becomes our bodies. We are alive because It is alive. It is defined by its relationships, as we are defined by the relationships of the 30 trillion cells that comprise every adult human body... their relationships are harmonious... they are love – compassionate, creative love. No two of us are alike. There is no divine hierarchical order separating human beings. Each one of us is a once – told tale, a once – sung song, a once – written novel, a once – read a poem, a once – danced dance... please tell me your tale; sing me your song; read me your novel; read me your poem; and dance me your dance. You honor me.

We have evidence in the cave drawings of what can well be said to be revelation of The Source because they are graphic representations of our curiosity about the Mystery. They go back 30,000 years. It was not until about 2,500 years ago that we developed writing, relying on the environment of a campfire to tell the stories of the tribe including its mystery stories. And let's be clear about this: the Judeo – Christian – Islamic Bible is full of mystery stories... and that is just great.

I consider it to be tragically naïve to assume that The Source stopped revealing Itself to us humans two and a half centuries ago. Why in the name of all that is holy would such behavior ever occur? Might it just be that we human beings – at least the children of Abraham – believe that revelation stopped when we stole the fruit of the Tree of Knowledge from The Source. To my way of thinking – today – I cannot believe that The Source would deny Its holy children anything of Itself. Rather, I believe that revelation is essential to the evolution of The Source, Itself! For me, therefore, Albert Einstein's fascinating theories of relativity, Beethoven's Fifth Symphony, and the Hubble telescope are all a part of the ongoing revelation necessary for the evolution.

We have only been able to understand that the whole universe has been evolving since the first spectrographs of stars came into the hands of Edwin Hubble in 1929. Albert Einstein saw in his general theory of relativity that the universe was not static and it stunned his belief systems so he modified it so the universe would be static. Hubble saw what Einstein had done and called him out for it. Einstein admitted to "the greatest blunder" he ever made in his life and corrected his mistakes What are the implications of that discovery? This has occupied the minds of brilliant people the world over ever since... not just a few, but millions of brilliant people – people who have access to the creativity of human minds as manifest in measuring equipment that can chase down the implications of Hubble's 1929 discovery. The greatest implication is that evolution is a fundamental quality and function of the whole universe

We now know that we are not accidents of a blind struggle for survival. We have not stolen knowledge; rather, it was given to us without condition. This empowers us to accrue experience, which, in turn, shows us that, in our perceived shame for having stolen knowledge from its Source, we have trudged out into an ever-deepening darkness *of our own choice*. Today, more than ever before, we are slowing down the trudge and raising our heads to see that the fading flickering light which illuminates our way comes from behind us. We are choosing to reverse course and go to the light that comes from our Source – a beacon calling us home – certain that Its direction gives us the power of peace that will take us to the stars in service of Source, Itself.

In this way, too, the legacy that became H.O.P.E. over the last 70 years becomes, in turn, a legacy that helps us move forward through a deep forest of darkness to the light that shows us the way Home. H.O.P.E. chooses to participate in *our* metamorphosis.

Notes

[i] Aleph is a mysterious, spiritual term that I have been attracted to because of the mysterious things have happened in my life that have no logical explanation. Spiritually and mystically, aleph contains all numbers and dimensions in the universe. Paolo Coelho wrote *Aleph*, (Knopf, September 2011) an autobiographical account of a trans-Siberian rail journey that described a mystical, dimensionless relationship with another person.

[ii]Lewisian Gneiss (Complex)" A major division of Precambrian rocks in northwestern Scotland Encyclopædia Britannica. Ultimate Reference Suite. Chicago: Encyclopædia Britannica, 2020.

[iii] Hysterectomy, surgical removal of the uterus, was then the only treatment for Gordon's hemorrhaging.

[iv] *A Course in Miracles*. Farmingdale, NY: Foundation for Inner Peace, 1975

[v] Eliade, Mircea, *Shamanism*. Princeton: Princeton University Press, 1972

[vi] Harner, Michael, PhD. *The Way of the Shaman*. San Francisco: Harper, 1990

[vii] In Gaelic, *anam cara*... O'Donohue, John. *Anam Cara, a Book of Celtic Wisdom*. New York: HarperCollins, 1997

[viii] Frankl, Viktor E., *Man's Search for Meaning*. New York: Pocket Books, 1985. In Dachau and three other concentration camps from 1942 to 1945, Frankl discovered that having a purpose to live for made survival possible.

[ix] Nightingale and Lloyd Victor Conant co-founded the Nightingale-Conant Corporation, 1400 South Wolf Road Bldg 300, Suite 103,Wheeling, IL 60090, to offer high quality, engaging instructional audio and video self-development media.

[x] The power of being able to choose attitudes is reflected in the statements of two famous physicians, William James M.D. (1842-1910), and Viktor Frankl, M.D. (1905-1997). James, founder of the school of pragmatism and the psychological movement of functionalism, said, "The greatest discovery of my generation is that human beings, by changing the inner attitudes of their minds, can change the outer aspects of their lives. It is too bad that more people will not accept this tremendous discovery and begin living it." Frankl, survivor of three years in four of the infamous Nazi concentration camps and originator of the psychotherapeutic process called *logotherapy*, said, "The last of the human freedoms is to choose one's attitude in a given set of circumstances; to choose one's way. It is this spiritual freedom that cannot be taken away that makes life meaningful and purposeful." (I wrote these words down at least 30 years ago as I listened to one of Nightingale's monthly *INSIGHT* tapes. Today, I have over 250 of these tapes, and have not the slightest idea in which one either quote can be found.)

[xi] Earl made it sound easy, but then he had only been working on developing his own attitudes of the mind since 1933, when he began a life-long study of the lives and methods of successful people. When he encountered the work of Napoleon Hill in 1950, he was able to develop a three-part *gift* for all humans. It comprised a formula, "We become what we think about;" a gold mine that made the formula work, the *mind*; and a key to access the gold mine, one's *attitude*.

[xii] The offerings of the Nightingale-Conant catalog today include the work of virtually every well-known person in the field of personal growth and development. I mention these five men because I connected with them when I first started tapping into the Nightingale-Conant resources.

[xiii] The title of a collection of his radio broadcasts and essays published in both audiotape and book form several years after Earl died in 1989.

[xiv] My teacher attributed this psychology to Karen Horney, a student of Freud, who came to the United States in 1932, and became one of the founders of the Association for the Advancement of Psychoanalysis and the American Institute for Psychoanalysis in 1942.

[xv] These educational groups for those newly diagnosed with cancer are a valuable service offered in most hospitals by the hospitals and the American Cancer Society.

[xvi] Sharon has been in many different areas of this country doing what she loves to do. We still stay in touch, and she knows why her name is the first name in the list of acknowledgments.

[xvii]http://peterkingsley.org/product/the-great-secret/

[xviii] These stories, except for mine, have all been published before and they are used here with the author's permission.

[xix] http://peterkingsley.org/wp-content/uploads/KingsleysLonging.pdf

www.ingramcontent.com/pod-product-compliance
Lightning Source LLC
Chambersburg PA
CBHW030026290326
41934CB00005B/500